Disorders of Menstruation

Disorders of Menstruation

EDITED BY

Paul B. Marshburn MD

Director of Reproductive Endocrinology and Infertility
Division of Reproductive Endocrinology and Infertility,
Department of Obstetrics and Gynecology,
Carolinas Medical Center,
Charlotte, North Carolina, USA

Bradley S. Hurst MD

Director, Program for Assisted Reproduction
Division of Reproductive Endocrinology and Infertility,
Department of Obstetrics and Gynecology,
Carolinas Medical Center,
Charlotte, North Carolina, USA

WILEY-BLACKWELL
A John Wiley & Sons, Ltd., Publication

This edition first published 2011, ® 2011 by Blackwell Publishing Ltd

Blackwell Publishing was acquired by John Wiley & Sons in February 2007. Blackwell's publishing program has been merged with Wiley's global Scientific, Technical and Medical business to form Wiley-Blackwell.

Registered office: John Wiley & Sons Ltd, The Atrium, Southern Gate, Chichester, West Sussex, PO19 8SQ, UK

Editorial offices: 9600 Garsington Road, Oxford, OX4 2DQ, UK
    The Atrium, Southern Gate, Chichester, West Sussex, PO19 8SQ, UK
    111 River Street, Hoboken, NJ 07030-5774, USA

For details of our global editorial offices, for customer services and for information about how to apply for permission to reuse the copyright material in this book please see our website at www.wiley.com/wiley-blackwell

The right of the author to be identified as the author of this work has been asserted in accordance with the UK Copyright, Designs and Patents Act 1988.

Wiley also publishes its books in a variety of electronic formats. Some content that appears in print may not be available in electronic books.

Designations used by companies to distinguish their products are often claimed as trademarks. All brand names and product names used in this book are trade names, service marks, trademarks or registered trademarks of their respective owners. The publisher is not associated with any product or vendor mentioned in this book. This publication is designed to provide accurate and authoritative information in regard to the subject matter covered. It is sold on the understanding that the publisher is not engaged in rendering professional services. If professional advice or other expert assistance is required, the services of a competent professional should be sought.

The contents of this work are intended to further general scientific research, understanding, and discussion only and are not intended and should not be relied upon as recommending or promoting a specific method, diagnosis, or treatment by physicians for any particular patient. The publisher and the author make no representations or warranties with respect to the accuracy or completeness of the contents of this work and specifically disclaim all warranties, including without limitation any implied warranties of fitness for a particular purpose. In view of ongoing research, equipment modifications, changes in governmental regulations, and the constant flow of information relating to the use of medicines, equipment, and devices, the reader is urged to review and evaluate the information provided in the package insert or instructions for each medicine, equipment, or device for, among other things, any changes in the instructions or indication of usage and for added warnings and precautions. Readers should consult with a specialist where appropriate. The fact that an organization or Website is referred to in this work as a citation and/or a potential source of further information does not mean that the author or the publisher endorses the information the organization or Website may provide or recommendations it may make. Further, readers should be aware that Internet Websites listed in this work may have changed or disappeared between when this work was written and when it is read. No warranty may be created or extended by any promotional statements for this work. Neither the publisher nor the author shall be liable for any damages arising herefrom.

Library of Congress Cataloging-in-Publication Data
Disorders of menstruation / edited by Paul B. Marshburn, Bradley S. Hurst.
    p. ; cm. – (Gynecology in practice)
  Includes bibliographical references and index.
  ISBN 978-1-4443-3277-3 (pbk. : alk. paper)
  1. Menstruation disorders.   I. Marshburn, Paul B.   II. Hurst, Bradley S.   III. Series: Gynecology in practice.
  [DNLM: 1. Menstruation Disturbances–pathology.   2. Menstrual Cycle–physiology. WP 550]
  RG161.D57 2011
  618.1'72–dc22
                          2010036449

A catalogue record for this book is available from the British Library.

This book is published in the following electronic formats: ePDF 9781444391800; Wiley Online Library 9781444391824; ePub 9781444391817

Set in 8.75/11.75 pt Utopia by Toppan Best-set Premedia Limited
Printed and bound in Malaysia by Vivar Printing Sdn Bhd

01   2011

Contents

Colour plate section can be found facing page 88.

Series Foreword

In recent decades, massive advances in medical science and technology have caused an explosion of information available to the practitioner. In the modern information age, it is not unusual for physicians to have a computer in their offices with the capability of accessing medical databases and literature searches. On the other hand, however, there is always a need for concise, readable, and highly practicable written resources. The purpose of this series is to fulfill this need in the field of gynecology.

The *Gynecology in Practice* series aims to present practical clinical guidance on effective patient care for the busy gynecologist. The goal of each volume is to provide an evidence-based approach for specific gynecologic problems. "Evidence at a glance" features in the text provide summaries of key trials or landmark papers that guide practice, and a selected bibliography at the end of each chapter provides a springboard for deeper reading. Even with a practical approach, it is important to review the crucial basic science necessary for effective diagnosis and management. This is reinforced by "Science revisited" boxes that remind readers of crucial anatomic, physiologic or pharmacologic principles for practice.

Each volume is edited by outstanding international experts who have brought together truly gifted clinicians to address many relevant clinical questions in their chapters. The first volumes in the series are on *Chronic Pelvic Pain*, one of the most challenging problems in gynecology, *Disorders of Menstruation*, *Infertility*, and *Contraception*. These will be followed by volumes on *Sexually Transmitted Diseases*, *Menopause*, *Urinary Incontinence*, *Endoscopic Surgeries*, and *Fibroids*, to name a few. I would like to express my gratitude to all the editors and authors, who, despite their other responsibilities, have contributed their time, effort, and expertise to this series.

Finally, I greatly appreciate the support of the staff at Wiley-Blackwell for their outstanding editorial competence. My special thanks go to Martin Sugden, PhD; without his vision and perseverance, this series would not have come to life. My sincere hope is that this novel and exciting series will serve women and their physicians well, and will be part of the diagnostic and therapeutic armamentarium of practicing gynecologists.

Aydin Arici, MD
Professor
Department of Obstetrics, Gynecology, and
Reproductive Sciences
Yale University School of Medicine
New Haven, USA

Dedications

This book is dedicated to my wife Nancy and my sons Aaron and Jonathan.

I owe a great debt to my mentors for their instruction, guidance, and inspiration. These leaders include: Arthur "Cap" Haney, Charles B. Hammond, Bruce R. Carr, Paul C. MacDonald, and Wallace C. Nunley, Jr.

I am grateful to Aydin Arici for the opportunity to edit this book and for the example of his intelligence and inquisitive nature.

Paul B. Marshburn, M.D.

I have been fortunate to work with many of the leaders in obstetrics, gynecology and reproductive endocrinology during my career. My approach to medicine, surgery, patient care, and teaching has been profoundly influenced by each, beginning with my brilliant and inspirational mentor in medical school, Dr. Griff Ross. As important as these have been in shaping my career, my wife Linda has helped me immeasurably and unwaveringly since college. I dedicate this book to my wife, mentors, friends, and family, including my beautiful daughters Kelly and Lisa. All have enriched my life and career.

Bradley S. Hurst, M.D.

Contributors

Karen D. Bradshaw, MD, Strauss Chair in Women's Health and Medical Director of the Lowe Foundation Center for Women's Preventative Healthcare, Division of Reproductive Endocrinology, Department of Obstetrics and Gynecology, University of Texas Southwestern Medical Center at Dallas, Dallas, Texas, USA

Isiah D. Harris, MD, Instructor and Clinical Fellow, Advanced Reproductive Medicine, University of Colorado Health Sciences Center, Aurora, Colorado, USA

Jennifer Kulp, MD, Clinical Instructor and Fellow in Obstetrics and Gynecology, Division of Reproductive Endocrinology, Yale University School of Medicine, New Haven, Connecticut, USA

Preeti P. Matkins, MD, Director of Child Maltreatment, Department of Pediatrics, Levine Children's Hospital at Carolinas Medical Center, Teen Health Connection, Charlotte, North Carolina, USA

Michelle L. Matthews, MD, Associate Director, Reproductive Endocrinology, Department of Obstetrics and Gynecology, Carolinas Medical Center, Charlotte, North Carolina, USA

Paul B. Miller, MD, Director of In Vitro Fertilization, Division of Reproductive Endocrinology and Infertility, University Medical Group, Greenville Hospital System, Greenville, South Carolina; GHS Associate Professor of Clinical Obstetrics and Gynecology, University of South Carolina Medical School, Columbia, South Carolina, USA

Kristin M. Rager, MD, MPH, Director of Adolescent Medicine, Department of Pediatrics, Levine Children's Hospital at Carolinas Medical Center, Teen Health Connection, Charlotte, North Carolina, USA

William D. Schlaff, MD, Professor and Director of Reproductive Endocrinology, University of Colorado Health Sciences Center, Aurora, Colorado, USA

David Tait, MD, Associate Director, Division of Gynecologic Oncology, Department of Obstetrics and Gynecology, Carolinas Medical Center, Charlotte, North Carolina, USA

Rebecca S. Usadi, MD, Associate Director, Reproductive Endocrinology and Infertility, Division of Reproductive Endocrinology and Infertility, Department of Obstetrics and Gynecology, Carolinas Medical Center, Charlotte, North Carolina, USA

Tara M. Vick, MD, Director of Ambulatory Care, Division of Obstetrics and Gynecology, Carolinas Medical Center, Charlotte, North Carolina, USA

Overview: Disorders of Menstruation

Paul B. Marshburn and Bradley S. Hurst

Carolinas Medical Center, Charlotte, North Carolina, USA

Introduction

This book is dedicated to the concept that menstrual cycle events are a *vital sign* for women. Irregularity in the pattern and amount of vaginal bleeding of uterine origin are often a sign of pathology or an aberration in the function of the hypothalamic, pituitary, and ovarian axis. Clues to disease states are afforded by changes in symptoms related to timing during the menstrual cycle. The process of menstruation may be accompanied by distressing symptoms such as menorrhagia (excessive menstrual blood loss), dysmenorrhea (painful periods), or oligoamenorrhea (infrequent or absent periods). When the menstrual vital sign is appropriately and methodically interpreted, it can provide a window into the diagnosis of conditions that might be life-threatening or herald systemic disorders that only secondarily impact menstrual function.

In the logical approach to disorders of menstruation, the astute clinician should employ the precepts of Bayes theorem. The medical application of this theorem is summarized by stating that the probability of diagnosing a clinical disorder depends upon evaluating historical and diagnostic information *in the population at risk*. It is obvious that the interpretation of cyclic menses in a 5-year-old girl is different from that of the cyclic pattern of vaginal bleeding in a woman of reproductive age. For this reason, we have organized this book to discuss disorders of menstruation in the chronologic order of the seasons of a woman's life. Therefore, sequential chapters begin with discussing abnormal vaginal bleeding in female infants and girls, followed by bleeding in peripubertal adolescents, women of reproductive age, those in the menopausal transition, and finally postmenopausal women. The likelihood of making an accurate diagnosis or achieving successful treatment is therefore dependent upon applying approaches in the appropriate age group and clinical setting, and in the population at risk.

This book is written for any practicing clinician who provides healthcare for girls and women. The authors have attempted to apply their knowledge to provide a conceptual framework to understand the mechanisms responsible for abnormal menstrual bleeding or early pregnancy failure. The exhaustive, academic presentation, however, is substituted for the direct and sensible approaches of expert authors who have a wealth of successful clinical experience based upon the rigorous evaluation of clinical trials. This clinically focused book is aimed at providing gynecologists in practice or in training with a guide for use "in the office" or "at the bedside." Our emphasis is upon providing an accurate diagnostic algorithm that leads to evidence-based therapy with approaches that are practical, efficient, and cost-effective.

Disorders of Menstruation, 1st edition. Edited by Paul B. Marshburn and Bradley S. Hurst.
© 2011 Blackwell Publishing Ltd.

Physiology of menstruation

The functional development of the endometrium is orchestrated by ovarian estrogen stimulation during the follicular phase, followed by the postovulatory influence of estrogen and progesterone from the corpus luteum to induce secretory endometrial transformation. This process is crucial for the perpetuation of the human species by inducing proper endometrial development for embryo implantation (Figure 1.1).

In the absence of embryo implantation, the endometrium is sloughed during menstruation or "the period," appropriately termed because it implies a beginning, a middle, and an end. Such a period occurs as a result of physiologic endometrial changes prompted by a decline in steroid production by the corpus luteum if pregnancy is not established. Regular, monthly, menstrual bleeding is the outward manifestation of the ovarian cycle that results from ovulation.

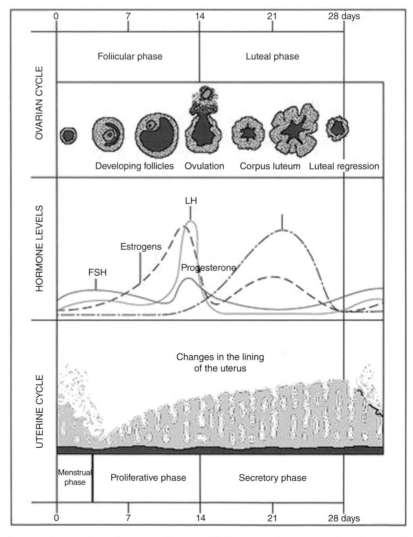

Figure 1.1 The ovarian cycle and its correlation with hormonal events and endometrial development during the menstrual cycle. FSH, follicle-stimulating hormone; LH, luteinizing hormone.

The landmark work of J. E. Markee, published in 1940, has been critical to the understanding of physiologic changes in primate endometrium during the menstrual cycle. Markee transplanted endometrium into an in-vivo observation chamber, the anterior chamber of the eye in rhesus monkeys. In this way, he directly observed endometrial changes during all the phases of the menstrual cycle in experiments that spanned 9 years of work. The cumulative studies of Markee and other investigators indicate that the process of menstruation is a series of *universal* endometrial events. Further investigation showed that the physiologic processes that start menstruation are also responsible for stopping it.

Paracrine factors, induced by the simultaneous decline in estradiol and progesterone, promote rhythmic contraction of the endometrial spiral arterioles. The resultant endometrial ischemia causes destabilization of the lysosomes, which release prostaglandins (primarily PGF2-alpha) that promote myometrial contractions. Fluid from the ischemic, liquefactive necrosis of endometrial tissue and blood is expelled by these myometrial contractions. Menstrual bleeding decreases after hemostasis from a combination of myometrial contractions and platelet plugging on exposed arteriolar type 2 collagen. The cessation of menstrual flow is completed with the initiation of endometrial tissue repair, growth, and angiogenesis that is required for preparation for implantation in the next cycle. Thus, a period of menstrual bleeding occurs through a process that is initiated by physiologic events that leads to its own conclusion.

Menstrual parameters

The menstrual cycle may be defined by its length, regularity, frequency, and pattern of menstrual blood loss. The average menstrual cycle length in the reproductive years is between 28 and 30 days, with an average period of menstruation of 4 days, and a volume of blood loss of approximately 30 mL. The primitive woman had fewer menstrual periods because the absence of contraceptive options meant that women were more often pregnant or lactating. Today, women experience approximately 400 menstrual cycles. It has been postulated that the development of hormonal contraception, methods of permanent sterilization, fewer pregnancies per woman, reduced intervals of lactational amenorrhea, and later age at time of first conception have all contributed to an increase in the number of menstrual cycles and the magnitude of menstrual disorders. Heavy menstrual and intermenstrual bleeding is the most common indication for hysterectomy and accounts for 4% of physician consultations annually.

"Abnormal uterine bleeding" is a term applied to deviations from the normal menstrual parameters defined above. The terminology used to describe "abnormal" menstruation, however, has not been defined in a universally accepted manner. The main causes of abnormal uterine bleeding are listed in Table 1.1. Benign disorders of the uterus may present with the complaint of excessive menstrual blood loss and/or an associated irregularity in the pattern of menstrual bleeding. Such benign disorders include endometrial polyps, fibroids, and adenomyosis. However, the vast majority of women complaining of excessive menstrual blood loss have normal endometrium.

The initial step in the evaluation of menstrual disorders involves differentiation between abnormal uterine bleeding caused by ovulatory dysfunction and bleeding secondary to genital lesions or systemic disease states. "Dysfunctional uterine bleeding" is a term that has been applied to abnormal uterine bleeding from irregular or absent ovulation. Dysfunctional uterine bleeding is a diagnosis of exclusion after determining that organic causes are not involved. Organic causes for abnormal uterine bleeding, exclusive of pregnancy-related bleeding, may be classified into three categories: pelvic pathology, systemic disease, and iatrogenic causes. If these organic causes can be excluded, ovulatory disorders are the likely cause of abnormal uterine bleeding.

Anovulatory bleeding is most commonly encountered at the beginning and end of the

Table 1.1 The main recognized causes of abnormal uterine bleeding

Pelvic pathology
Uterine leiomyomas
Uterine adenomyomas or diffuse adenomyosis
Endometrial polyps
Endometrial hyperplasia
Endometrial adenocarcinoma, rare sarcomas
Uterine or cervical infection
Endometrial or cervical infections
Benign cervical disease
Cervical squamous and adenocarcinoma
Myometrial hypertrophy
Uterine arteriovenous malformations (complications of unrecognized early pregnancy)
Systemic disease
Disorders of hemostasis (typically von Willebrand disease and platelet disorders, excessive
   anticoagulation)
Hypothyroidism
Other rarities such as systemic lupus erythematosus and chronic liver failure
Dysfunctional uterine bleeding (DUB)
Ovulatory DUB—a primary endometrial disorder of the molecular mechanisms controlling the
   volume of blood lost during menstruation
Anovulatory DUB—a primary disorder of the hypothalamic–pituitary–ovarian axis resulting
in excessive unopposed ovarian estrogen secretion and a secondary endometrial disturbance

Reproduced from Woolcock et al., 2008, with permission.

reproductive years. The immaturity of the hypothalamic–pituitary–ovarian axis causes infrequent ovulation and irregular uterine bleeding in the peripubertal years, while irregular bleeding during the menopausal transition is encountered with the oocyte depletion of diminishing ovarian reserve.

The World Health Organization (WHO) proposed a practical classification for disorders of ovulation. The WHO designated three groups (I, II, III) based on the state of gonadotropin and estrogen secretion. The diagnosis of hypogonadotropic (low luteinizing hormone [LH] and follicle-stimulating hormone [FSH]) and hypoestrogenic anovulation (WHO group I) is often referred to as hypothalamic anovulation. The WHO group I disorders result from a variety of stressors or primary disease states that impact the hypothalamus to alter gonadotropin-releasing hormone (GnRH) pulsatility, with disruption of cyclic gonadotropin release. Hypothalamic anovulation may result from a congenital disorder of formation of the neurons

that secrete GnRH, but also could be secondary to organic lesions of the brain or stress from psychological or other disease states.

Hypergonadotropic anovulation (WHO group III; high LH and FSH) is related to follicle and oocyte depletion. This grouping comprises women who naturally proceed through the transition to menopause, but also includes women who exhibit primary or secondary ovarian insufficiency, a category often referred to as premature ovarian failure.

The most problematic group of anovulatory disorders to define, however, is WHO group II, the so-called normogonadotropic, normoestrogenic cases. WHO group II, which constitutes by far the largest group of patients, is composed of a variety of hormonal abnormalities, with the largest category representing the polycystic ovarian syndrome (PCOS). The heterogeneity of this group prevents a single unified approach to the diagnosis of specific disorders within the WHO group II designation. Obesity, adrenal and thyroid dysfunction, and particular metabolic diseases can cause inappropriate extragonadal production of estrogen and androgen. This status can "short-circuit" the normal sex steroid feedback mechanism to the hypothalamus and pituitary because inappropriate extragonadal production of estrogen and androgen will produce tonic suppression of the cyclic LH and FSH secretion necessary for ovulation. Therefore, a woman can have a variety of causes for normogonadotropic, normoestrogenic anovulation (WHO group II), and these causes are not elucidated by the measurement of serum estradiol, FSH, and LH. For appropriate management of these patients, the astute diagnostician must carefully solicit pertinent historical information and carefully observe cutaneous, genital, and constitutional signs associated with both normal and abnormal estrogen and androgen production.

Organization of the book

Disorders of Menstruation is a clinical reference for the medical management of the female with abnormal vaginal bleeding. The chapters are organized sequentially in a chronology from infancy to old age throughout a woman's life. A given sign, symptom, or finding within a particular age group will often have markedly different health implications. Because the myriad causes of disordered menstruation often have a unique presentation in each age group, there is an intentional overlap of information among chapters to discuss these important distinctions.

The working assumption in this reference is that readers will be looking for advice and information that will assist them in clinical encounters, without overemphasis on the theoretical aspects of approaches and procedures. The authors, however, understand the importance of reviewing the crucial basic science necessary for effective diagnosis and management. The chapters are not heavily referenced, but citations of important reviews and major contributions are provided in the "Selected bibliography" at the end of each chapter.

Information is provided in a format that makes reading easier and allows the busy clinician to quickly access the essential information for patient care. Practical guidance to readers will be provided through the use of algorithms and guidelines where they are appropriate. Key evi-dence (clinical trials, Cochrane Database citations, other meta-analyses) is summarized in "Evidence at a glance" boxes. "Tips and tricks" boxes provide hints on improving outcomes by indicating practical techniques, pertinent patient questioning, or pertinent signs or symptoms that direct clinical management. The clinical tips may be derived from experience rather than formal evidence, but a rationale is provided to support suggested practices. "Caution" warning boxes suggest hints on avoiding problems, perhaps via a statement of contraindications or by warning of pitfalls in management. "Science revisited" boxes reveal a quick and clear reminder of the basic science principles necessary for understanding principles of practice.

Orientation to the chapters

Vaginal bleeding in the prepubertal infant and girl signifies an abnormality that demands prompt investigation. Chapter 2, entitled "Prepubertal Genital Bleeding," defines the best approaches for management of the pediatric population, who often cannot provide a clear history and may be threatened by a sensitive examination. The authors provide a clear and detailed approach to the pertinent gynecologic history and examination of the female child. Their defined approach maximizes the opportunities to make an "office" diagnosis. These clinicians indicate that most causes of prepubertal genital bleeding include trauma, intravaginal foreign bodies, infection, and vulvovaginal dermatologic disorders. Indications of sexual abuse must be confirmed, and the authors emphasize the means to fulfill the legal mandate that clinicians report these incidents to authorities for child protection. The malignant causes of prepubertal genital bleeding are then presented, with specific indications for making a prompt diagnosis and referral. Precocious puberty may present with vaginal bleeding in the pediatric age group. In this case, other signs of premature pubertal progress are seen, which may include the early development of the breasts, axillary and pubic hair, and a growth spurt with associated advanced bone maturation. The details of diagnosis and management of precocious puberty are explored in depth in the next chapter.

Chapter 3, on "Irregular Vaginal Bleeding and Amenorrhea During the Pubertal Years," provides a comprehensive overview of the normal pubertal milestones and highlights boundaries for when deviation from the normal sequence of female development is a cause for concern. The causes of precocious puberty are first delineated so the diagnosing physician will be armed with the most common elements of the differential diagnosis. This is followed by a direct and practical diagnostic approach that helps in understanding how historical, physical examination, and laboratory findings will allow categorization of the differential causes of precocious puberty into central (above the neck) or peripheral (below the neck) abnormalities. Precocious puberty signifies the potential for serious health and reproductive consequences. The wealth of practical knowledge revealed in this chapter will assist the clinician in the most efficient and accurate method to best manage this emotionally charged situation.

If puberty is delayed, young women and parents need education about whether this condition is within the normal physiologic range of development or whether this represents a condition of primary amenorrhea. The differential diagnosis for primary amenorrhea has significantly different implications when compared to the absence of periods once puberty is complete and menstruation has started (secondary amenorrhea). While certain presenting signs will immediately clue the physician to the origin of the cause of primary amenorrhea (e.g., Turner's syndrome, müllerian agenesis, androgen insensitivity), other causes are not obvious, and their diagnosis requires a systematic management algorithm that is clearly presented in this chapter.

Menarche heralds the transition from childhood to the reproductively competent woman. Adolescents and their parents, however, are often unsure about what represents normal menstrual patterns after menarche. For the first 18 months after menarche, irregular menstrual bleeding from infrequent ovulation is common. Rarely, however, should the time interval between cycles be greater than 90 days. Amenorrhea for greater than 3 months or menstrual flow for longer than 7 days is abnormal in the adolescent. In these cases, adolescents should be evaluated in order to detect conditions such as eating disorders, PCOS, von Willebrand disease, or other anatomic abnormalities of the female genital tract. The American College of Obstetricians and Gynecologists recommends that the initial visit to an obstetrician-gynecologist should take place around age 13–15 to discuss preventative services, health guidance about adolescent physical development, expectations for menstrual cyclicity, and menstrual hygiene.

Menstrual disorders are common during the reproductive years, and the central chapters of this book define the parameters for physiologic and abnormal vaginal bleeding. Chapter 4, entitled "Menstrual Disorders During the Reproductive Years," comprehensively introduces and orients the clinician to general points of management. Emphasis is placed upon the goal of differentiating whether the cause is related to disordered ovulation secondary to reproductive or systemic disease or to an anatomic abnormality from a woman's genital organs. Iatrogenic causes and pregnancy-related bleeding are common, and these factors should be considered first before healthcare providers initiate diagnostic testing.

Hyperandrogenic ovulatory dysfunction, or PCOS, is the most common endocrine disorder of reproductive-aged women. Chapter 5, entitled "Abnormal Menstrual Bleeding in Hyperandrogenic Ovulatory Dysfunction," is devoted entirely to the care of these women because the clinician plays a critical role not only towards insuring both general and reproductive health, but also in excluding other serious endocrine disorders that masquerade as PCOS. The emergence of PCOS occurs in adolescence, and its cause is not yet understood. A hallmark of the metabolic consequences of PCOS is its association with insulin resistance, which increases the risk of adult-onset diabetes and premature atherosclerotic heart disease. This chapter reviews the common clinical presentations, etiology, and diagnostic evaluation of hyperandrogenic ovulatory disorders. A discussion of treatment highlights the most effective methods for the regulation of menstrual function, prevention of endometrial cancer, and correction of ovulatory dysfunction for fertility. Practical pearls of advice are given to most effectively and safely implement weight reduction for women with PCOS, which helps to prevent adult-onset diabetes and reverse the harmful impact of unchecked metabolic syndrome. Modern options for managing the negative cosmetic consequences of hyperandrogenism are also presented.

The anatomic or mechanical causes of excessive uterine bleeding represent one of the most common reasons that a woman will seek the care of her gynecologist.

Chapters 6 and 7, entitled, "Abnormal Uterine Bleeding due to Anatomic Causes: Diagnosis" and "Abnormal Uterine Bleeding due to Anatomic Causes: Treatment" address these essential issues of reproductive-aged women. Too frequently, the option offered for the management of such abnormal uterine bleeding is hysterectomy. Often the presence of benign uterine neoplasms, such as polyps and leiomyomas (fibroids), prompts even the most careful clinician to incorrectly assume that the tumor is the direct cause for abnormal bleeding. The diagnostic algorithm presented represents a thoughtful and complete consideration of coexistent factors and the nuances of conservative management. This chapter initially reveals the details of how to use the history, physical examination, and pelvic imaging to make an accurate diagnosis. Only then can all contributing factors be optimally addressed to correct the problem while minimizing invasiveness and the cost of treatment. Alternatives to hysterectomy include a number of new medical interventions and conservative surgical options that will correct the problem while allowing a woman to maintain her reproductive function. If pregnancy is not desired, however, excellent results can be achieved with options such as intrauterine progestin-releasing systems or endometrial ablation applied in an office setting.

The author's extensive surgical experience delivers a presentation of creative, minimally invasive surgical options that are afforded by novel approaches and new technology. Recommendations for best approaches are based upon a distillation of research and practical knowledge from clinical experience. The advantages and pitfalls of employing pre- and postoperative surgical adjuncts are critically evaluated. The author's goal is to enhance a patient's satisfaction with her care by allowing her to choose from all of the options to correct abnormal bleed-ing from anatomic causes. The approaches delineated in these chapters will enable the gynecologist to avoid hysterectomy when possible and to recommend it when indicated.

Chapter 8, entitled "Infrequent Menstrual Bleeding and Amenorrhea During the Reproductive Years," reveals that a different profile of reproductive hormone imbalances and anatomic abnormalities is encountered in reproductive-aged women with menstrual disorders when compared to adolescents with primary amenorrhea and abnormal uterine bleeding. Functional hypothalamic amenorrhea, prolactin-secreting adenomas, polycystic ovaries, and ovarian failure are included among the hormonal causes of secondary amenorrhea. Disease states such as exercise-induced hypothalamic amenorrhea and anorexia nervosa are associated with low concentrations of the appetite-regulating hormone leptin, and both present a similar spectrum of neuroendocrine abnormalities. The finding of premature ovarian insufficiency as a cause of secondary amenorrhea warrants an evaluation for polyglandular autoimmune dysfunction of the pancreas and the thyroid, parathyroid, and adrenal glands. Women with normal hormonal parameters may have anomalous genital tracts or intrauterine adhesions. A systematic approach to women with amenorrhea based on signs and symptoms will establish an accurate diagnosis in most cases, allowing effective treatment.

Normal ovarian function rather than reproductive endocrine imbalance is associated with menstrual cycle-related disorders. Chapter 9, entitled "Menstrual Cycle-related Clinical Disorders," discusses the medical conditions that appear or worsen during particular phases of the menstrual cycle to significantly impair the health of women. Cyclic fluctuation in estrogen and progesterone can alter cognitive and sensory processing, emotional wellbeing, appetite, and certain disease states in women. The diagnosis and modern management of premenstrual syndrome, menstrual migraine, catamenial epilepsy, and other medical conditions are discussed in this chapter. The accurate and prospective documentation of symptoms in relation to a particular phase of the menstrual cycle will help diagnose these cyclic disease states and provide a strategy for preventative and targeted therapeutic intervention. Details are provided for when to collaborate with medical consultants to provide the optimum outcome for patients.

The menopausal transition represents a time of great variability in reproductive hormone dynamics and menstrual cycle characteristics. In Chapter 10, entitled "Irregular Uterine Bleeding During the Menopausal Transition," the authors present the optimum methods for clinically evaluating when this transition begins and its impact on fertility and general health. Prior to detectable menstrual cycle changes, such as the gradual shortening of mean cycle length, a decline in the number of ovarian follicles may be evident by intermittent ovarian function and vasomotor symptoms. There is no period in a woman's life when unpredictable uterine bleeding occurs with greater frequency than during the menopausal transition. Thyroid dysfunction is commonly uncovered. When ovulatory dysfunction becomes evident, anatomic uterine causes should be sought, and the authors discuss the safe and appropriate hormonal and nonhormonal options to control irregular bleeding in these women. With waning ovulation in the menopausal transition, persistent endometrial exposure to estrogen without cyclic progesterone secretion can lead to hyperplasia and possibly endometrial adenocarcinoma.

Postmenopausal bleeding accounts for up to 10% of all gynecologic visits. The authors of Chapter 11, entitled "Postmenopausal Bleeding," point out that any vaginal bleeding in the menopause is abnormal and must be evaluated to insure that cancer is not the cause. Approximately 90% of postmenopausal bleeding, however, is associated with a benign condition, such as endometrial atrophy or polyps of the endocervix or endometrium. The incidence, clinical presentation, and systematic evaluation of the female genital cancers is presented to indicate the methods for detecting and treating neoplasia of the vulva, vagina, cervix, endometrium, myometrium, and fallopian tubes as a cause of postmenopausal bleeding. The authors present evidence supporting the approach that postmenopausal bleeding should initially be evaluated by transvaginal ultrasonography with an endometrial biopsy to follow if the endometrial thickness is greater than 4 mm. Saline infusion sonography and ultimately hysteroscopy with targeted biopsy of the endometrial cavity should be employed if such testing is not definitive. Hormone treatment is associated with abnormal bleeding in up to 40% of patients. The frequency of unplanned bleeding with sequential and continuous regimens of postmenopausal hormone therapy is reviewed. Systemic diseases and anticoagulant medications can cause postmenopausal bleeding and may be a sign requiring medical attention.

Summary

Menstrual cycle events can be seen to be a *vital sign* related to women's health, and the application of the approaches within this book will greatly aid healthcare providers who care for females of all ages. The ease of access to the clinical insights and the diagnostic and management algorithms herein will assist practitioners at the time of the clinic visit to use these principles to benefit the health of women in their care.

Selected bibliography

Chen BH, Guidice LC. Dysfunctional uterine bleeding. West J Med 1998;169:280–4.

Coulter A, McPherson K, Vessey M. Do British women undergo too many or too few hysterectomies? Soc Sci Med 1988;27:987–94.

Farquhar CM, Lethaby A, Sowter M, Verry J, Baranyi J. An evaluation for risk factors for endometrial hyperplasia in premenopausal women with abnormal menstrual bleeding. Am J Obstet Gynecol 1999;181:525–9.

Fraser IS, Inceboz US. Defining disturbances of the menstrual cycle. In: O'Brien S, Cameron I, MacLean A, eds. Disorders of the menstrual cycle. London: RCOG Press; 2000. pp. 141–52.

Markee JE. Menstruation in intraocular endometrial transplants in the rhesus monkey. Contr Embryol Carneg Inst 1940;28:219–308.

Rodgers WH, Matrisian LM, Giudice LC et al. Patterns of metalloproteinase expression in cycling endometrium imply differential functions and regulation by steroid hormones. J Clin Invest 1994;94:946–53.

Vuorento T, Huhtaniemi I. Daily levels of salivary progesterone during the menstrual cycle in adolescent girls. Fertil Steril 1992;58:685–90.

Woolcock JG, Critchley HO, Munro MG, Broder MS, Fraser IS. Review of the confusion in current and historical terminology and definitions for disturbances of menstrual bleeding. Fertil Steril 2008;90:2269–80.

World Health Organization Scientific Group. Agents stimulating gonadal function in the human. Report No. 514. Geneva: WHO; 1976.

2

Prepubertal Genital Bleeding

Kristin M. Rager, Preeti P. Matkins, and Tara M. Vick

Levine Children's Hospital at Carolinas Medical Center, Charlotte, North Carolina, USA

Introduction

Genital bleeding in a prepubertal female can be very frightening for both the girl and her parents. The role of the medical provider is not only to diagnose and treat the cause of the bleeding, but also to perform the appropriate examination in such a way that is least traumatic to all involved. There are many causes of prepubertal genital bleeding (Table 2.1). This chapter will review those causes, as well as describe physical examination positions and techniques.

Gynecologic history and physical examination

The best way to distinguish a normal from an abnormal pediatric gynecologic examination is to make the genital examination part of every physical examination. This enables the provider to become very familiar with variants of normal anatomy, and also removes the stigma associated with the genital examination for the patient. Parents readily accept this part of the examination as routine; especially when presented as a normal portion of a complete examination. Performing an external genitourinary examination on all female infants and girls during annual physicals is recommended by the American Academy of Pediatrics.

In the case of a genitourinary examination due to a concerning sign or symptom, a thorough history of the complaint should first be obtained.

In general, the history should include the time course of the complaint, how the concern arose, a description of any genital bleeding or discharge, pain or discomfort, as well as any treatments used prior to the visit. Any use of or exposure to medications, especially estrogen-containing substances, may be relevant. A female newborn infant may experience withdrawal vaginal bleeding as a result of disruption of maternal estrogen exposure *in utero*. Any exogenous estrogen exposure, such as estrogen-containing topical or oral medications may also cause estrogenization of the hymen and/or withdrawal vaginal bleeding. Close, skin-to-skin contact with a parent using topical creams or ointments containing estrogen or testosterone can be absorbed by the child and produce systemic effects. A history or observation of breast development, the presence of pubic or axillary hair, documented precocious growth spurts, or evidence of body odor should alert the physician to the possibility of precocious puberty (see Chapter 3). In the case of vaginal discharge or bleeding, it is best for the child *not* to have bathed for at least 24 hours prior to the examination.

Adolescents above the age of 11 should also have a history taken privately, that is, without the parent or guardian present. It is important to ask about sexual contact (intercourse, digital, oral, and anal sexual contact). It is very important to ask the age of the patient's sexual contacts. "Consensual" contact must also be viewed in the sense of compli-

Disorders of Menstruation, 1st edition. Edited by Paul B. Marshburn and Bradley S. Hurst.
© 2011 Blackwell Publishing Ltd.

Table 2.1 Causes of genital bleeding in preadolescent females

Unintentional trauma
Sexual abuse
Vulvovaginitis
Foreign bodies
Urethral prolapse
Lichen sclerosus et atrophicus
Pruritis/excoriations
Tumors
Precocious puberty

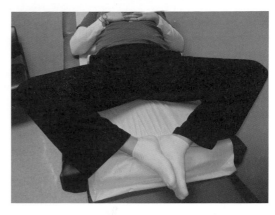

Figure 2.1 Examination positioning—frog-leg.

ant victims or non-forcible sexual assault. If there is concern about sexual abuse or assault, care should be taken when considering gathering forensic evidence and the medical care of the patient. Every state has differing laws on mandated reporting of child abuse, but all are clear that concern or suspicion of abuse requires reporting; proof of abuse is not required. A clinician should report to child protective services and/or local law enforcement in accordance with local laws. Reporting in good faith is protected by liability laws.

> **⚕ CAUTION**
>
> Providers must report ANY suspicion or concern of sexual abuse of minors to local authorities, regardless of the presence of any evidence or physical findings.

An external genital examination is almost always adequate. Occasionally, the use of saline irrigation may assist in separating tissue and improving visibility. In prepubertal girls, the hymen is exquisitely tender, and if vaginal samples are necessary, care should be taken not to touch the rim of the hymen. Use of a speculum is rarely indicated in prepubertal girls and should be reserved for occasions requiring anesthesia such as uncontrolled bleeding, an intravaginal foreign body with significant trauma, or serious fascial infections. In adolescents, the estrogenized hymen is not tender to touch with cotton swabs or even a balloon catheter (used for urinary catheterization). These catheters with a balloon tip can be filled after insertion into the vagina to help visualize the edges of the hymen.

Magnification for better visualization may be helpful. The use of various tools, including an otoscope, ophthalmoscope, or colposcope may be of assistance, but often is not required. A good light source is necessary and can be an overhead or floor light source or attached to a tool used for magnification. Some providers may use a digital camera for documentation.

There are three examination positions for performing gynecologic examinations in children/young adolescents. These include the frog-leg or butterfly position (Figure 2.1), the dorsal lithotomy position, and the knee–chest position (Figure 2.2). In the frog-leg position, the patient lies supine with her knees bent and her ankles brought towards her genital area (like a frog). In girls with longer legs, the dorsal lithotomy position may be more comfortable. In this position, the patient should have her buttocks close to the edge of the table. It may be useful to examine a child in the parent's lap if needed.

The third position used for examination is knee–chest. In this position, the child is placed on her knees, with her feet at the end of the examination table, and her head lying on her folded elbows. The knee–chest position is excellent for visualizing the posterior hymen and is very helpful if the examination in the frog-leg or dorsal lithotomy position reveals possible abnormalities in the posterior hymenal rim. This position may also be helpful in visualizing the vaginal

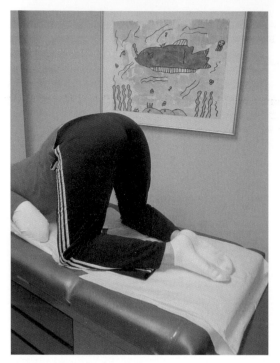

Figure 2.2 Examination positioning—knee–chest.

vault in cases of concern of a foreign body. Missing tissue in the posterior hymenal rim viewed in the frog-leg or dorsal lithotomy position may actually represent redundant tissue that is responding to gravity. A knee–chest examination is necessary to confirm tissue abnormalities versus gravity effects.

There are also three useful examination techniques: labial separation, labial traction, and buttock traction. Labial separation involves gentle separation of the labia majora at about half way along their length to visualize the hymenal orifice as well as the perilabial area, the clitoral hood and the urethral area. Labial traction involves gently grasping the labia majora and applying outward and downward traction. Care must be taken not to apply undue traction to the sensitive posterior commissure area. Any erythema or irritation of the vulvar area may result in pain, so pressure should be applied carefully. Buttock traction is used in the knee–chest position. The buttocks are lifted and separated to visualize the vulvar area, including the posterior hymenal rim. Again, be careful not to apply undue traction to the posterior commissure.

Documentation of the genital examination should include describing the technique and position utilized. Findings should be reported in a "clock" configuration, with 12 o'clock representing the urethra and 6 o'clock the posterior rim of the hymen when the patient is supine.

There are many hymenal variants (Figure 2.3). Hymenal appearance is affected by estrogen, which is present in the newborn period from in utero estrogen exposure and may persist until 2–3 years of age. Hymenal changes due to estrogen present again with onset of puberty.

Of note, the orifice diameter of the hymen is not an indication of previous trauma or injury. The orifice diameter of the hymen may depend upon multiple factors, including patient relaxation, healthcare provider's technique, and weight of the patient. Patient relaxation is very important in the genitourinary examination, and one should consider the time required to have a patient and parent comfortable with the examination. The use of blowing bubbles or reading books to relax the patient may be considered. If the patient is unable to relax to provide an adequate examination, the urgency should be considered. An emergent examination may require an evaluation under anesthesia; otherwise a repeat visit should be scheduled if the girl and/or parent are uncomfortable with the setting.

The focus of hymenal examination should be from 3 to 9 o'clock when the patient is supine. Abnormalities, including partial or complete transection of the hymen at 3–6 o'clock, should be confirmed in the knee–chest position. Hymenal abnormalities in the 3–6 o'clock position are very concerning for penetrating injury, including abuse. Again, it should be kept in mind

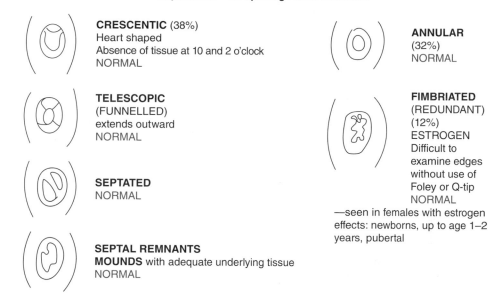

Hymenal types
frog-leg position
(percentage in prepubertal girls with no history of abuse)

Imperforate = no opening = NOT NORMAL

CRESCENTIC (38%)
Heart shaped
Absence of tissue at 10 and 2 o'clock
NORMAL

ANNULAR
(32%)
NORMAL

TELESCOPIC
(FUNNELLED)
extends outward
NORMAL

FIMBRIATED
(REDUNDANT)
(12%)
ESTROGEN
Difficult to
examine edges
without use of
Foley or Q-tip
NORMAL
—seen in females with estrogen
effects: newborns, up to age 1–2
years, pubertal

SEPTATED
NORMAL

SEPTAL REMNANTS
MOUNDS with adequate underlying tissue
NORMAL

Figure 2.3 Hymenal variants.

that the hymenal tissue is distensible, so penetration may not be evident as abnormalities on examination.

If, on taking the history, a persistent or recurrent discharge is described, or if on physical examination the discharge is purulent or grossly blood-tinged, vaginal swabs may be obtained for office evaluation of a wet mount preparation (saline and potassium hydroxide) and for laboratory culture analysis. Organisms for culture analysis are included in Table 2.2 (see next section). The swab should be premoistened with saline and carefully inserted into the vagina without touching the edges of the sensitive hymen. Run the swab against the lateral wall of the vagina to obtain a specimen. If the young girl is able to cooperate, ask her to cough at the time of the insertion of the swab. This will have the twofold effect of causing a distraction and allowing the hymen to open. Vaginal samples may also be acquired by vaginal lavage. A saline syringe may be attached to either a pediatric urethral catheter or a 14-gauge venous catheter (with the needle removed) to allow sample aspi-

ration or vaginal washings that can flow onto the specimen swabs. Topical lidocaine gel may be used as an anesthetic to aid in the collection or lavage.

After collecting the specimen swab, the applicator is first mixed with a drop of saline on a glass slide and then with a drop of 10% potassium hydroxide on a second slide. Cover slips are then placed, and the slides may be examined under low and high powers. In bacterial vaginosis, clue cells can be identified as bacterium-studded epithelial cells. Flagellated, motile organisms slightly larger than white blood cells may be identified as trichomonads. The potassium hydroxide slide may reveal budding pseudohyphae and yeast forms indicative of *Candida* yeast vaginitis. Touching the specimen swab to pH paper during the examination may be helpful in making a diagnosis. In prepubertal girls, the vaginal pH is neutral (6.5–7.5), providing an optimal environment for bacterial growth. In pubertal adolescent girls, the pH is acidic (less than 4.5). Bacterial vaginosis and *Trichomonas* vaginitis raise the normal pH to greater than 4.5.

Causes of prepubertal genital bleeding

Benign

Injuries to the vulvar and perivulvar area are relatively common in prepubertal girls and usually present with bleeding or dysuria. Generally, there is a history of trauma, although one should remember that playground or bicycle injuries may not be immediately recalled, especially if the child was in the care of others (daycare, school) at the time of the injury. Straddle injuries involve the vulvar and perivulvar area and may present as abrasions, lacerations, or bruising. The genital skin is very well vascularized and heals quickly. In general, treatment is symptomatic only, with use of barrier (petrolatum [petroleum] jelly) to protect the skin and decrease pain from contact with urine. Large lacerations may require suturing. Injuries to the vaginal orifice and hymen are less likely to be associated with straddle injuries. In cases where a girl has hymenal injuries attributed to a straddle injury, one should consider whether an impalement type of accidental injury has occurred and also consider possibility of inflicted injury/abuse.

Vulvovaginitis may present with a vulvar inflammation, vulvar pruritis, vaginal discharge, or vaginal bleeding. A wide range of normal vaginal flora can be cultured in girls without symptoms, including *Bacteroides*, *Staphylococcus*, and *Streptococcus* species, lactobacilli, diphtheroids, and Gram-negative enteric organisms, usually *Escherichia coli*. The vaginal culture from girls with vaginitis typically grows normal flora. The specific infections that occur in the prepubertal girl are typically respiratory, enteric, or sexually transmitted infections (Table 2.2). Vulvovaginitis due to these organisms may or may not present with concomitant respiratory or gastrointestinal illness. For example, *Shigella* infection can result in a mucopurulent, sometimes bloody vaginal discharge, but is associated with diarrhea in only approximately 25% of presentations. The most common respiratory organism to cause vaginitis is *Streptococcus pyogenes*

Table 2.2 Organisms implicated in prepubertal vulvovaginitis

Respiratory pathogens
Streptococcus pyogenes (group A beta-hemolytic *Streptococcus*)
Staphylococcus aureus
Haemophilus influenzae
Streptococcus pneumoniae
Moraxella catarrhalis
Neisseria meningitidis
Enteric pathogens
Shigella
Yersinia
Candida
Sexually transmitted infections
Neisseria gonorrhoeae
Chlamydia trachomatis
Trichomonas vaginalis
Herpes simplex virus
Condyloma acuminata (human papillomavirus)
Pinworms, other helminthes

(Group A beta-hemolytic *Streptococcus*). Although throat cultures frequently are positive, only 25–30% of patients have symptoms of pharyngitis. *Candida* vulvitis may be common in pubertal, estrogenized girls; however, it is not common in prepubertal girls unless there is an associated risk factor such as immunosuppression from diabetes. Empiric antibiotic therapy or directive treatment of the causative organism will result in a resolution of vaginal bleeding occurring due to vulvovaginitis.

A foreign body in the vagina may present with a foul-smelling, bloody discharge and is the etiology underlying a great majority of bleeding in young girls. The bleeding is described as either bright red or brown, light in amount, and usually appearing sporadically. It is uncommon for the girl to recall or reveal the history of a vaginal placement of a foreign object. In fact, the most common item is retained toilet paper. This is especially likely to occur during toilet training, as girls become increasingly responsible for their own post-void hygiene or "wiping." Other foreign bodies are not usually radio-opaque, so diagnosis requires an office examination or examination with sedation or under anesthesia. Toilet paper and other small objects may be removed with vaginal lavage as previously described. Other objects may be removed with forceps after appropriate sedation. The use of a hysteroscope or cystoscope may be necessary for adequate lavage and visualization. The intravaginal hysterosocopic evaluation for retained foreign bodies requires performance under anesthesia.

One of the most common causes of "vaginal bleeding" in the prepubertal female is not vaginal at all. Urethral prolapse often presents as sudden, painless genitourinary bleeding that may be described as profuse. There is no history of preceding trauma. On examination, in the supine position, there is an area of red swollen tissue that obscures visualization of genital landmarks. It may be difficult to distinguish the clitoral hood, hymenal orifice, and urethra. The protruding, swollen, erythematous tissue is very tender. To the inexperienced examiner, the findings may be very concerning for trauma or tumor. Careful examination will reveal that the area of concern that is obscuring normal structures is actually a

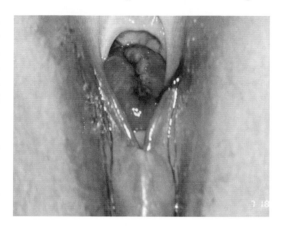

Figure 2.4 Urethral prolapse (see Plate 2.4).

prolapsed urethra. Knee–chest examination with buttock traction will often reveal a normal view of the posterior hymenal rim with an obvious urethral prolapse anteriorly (Figure 2.4).

Urethral prolapse occurs in hypoestrogenic states: postmenopausal women, and girls between toddler age and puberty. This condition is more common in African-American girls than Caucasian or Latina girls. Initial treatment is estrogen cream applied directly to the prolapsed area twice a day for 7–10 days. Parents should be instructed on direct administration. Sitz baths once or twice a day are recommended for comfort. If the patient has a history of constipation, stool softeners may be considered to reduce straining. If initial medical treatment fails or if the prolapse is strangulated (presenting with many areas of clotted tissue), consultation with a pediatric gynecologist or pediatric urologist should be considered for surgical repair.

Lichen sclerosus et atrophicus is an autoimmune condition that is most common in hypoestrogenic states such as menopause, but may present in prepubertal children. The presentation of this dermatologic condition is variable, with some girls presenting with painless genital bleeding, some with genital or vulvar pain or itching and labial bleeding, and some with concerns of labial trauma. The course may be indolent, with several waxing and waning episodes prior to diagnosis.

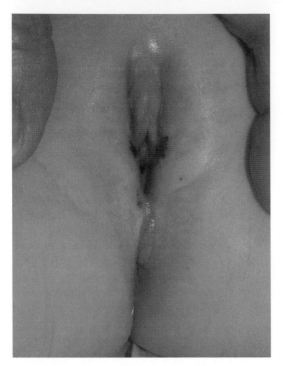

Figure 2.5 Lichen sclerosus et atrophicus (see Plate 2.5).

On examination, there is a hypopigmented, atrophic area, usually in an hourglass shape around the vulva and anus (Figure 2.5). This distribution may also be referred to as a "figure of eight." The introitus is not affected. Depending on the course of the condition at the time of the examination, thinned skin resulting in subepithelial bleeding (blood blisters) may be present. These areas of bleeding can be confused with trauma, either accidental or inflicted. Unlike a single episode of trauma, these areas may return after they have been considered healed. The condition may cause discomfort, and the inflammatory response may produce discharge from the affected areas. Again, careful examination and knowledge of normal anatomy is necessary in making an accurate diagnosis.

Treatment generally requires a medium- or high-potency steroid such as clobetasol (Temovate) 0.05% ointment. These topical steroid ointments can be prescribed for a short course to be used twice a day for 7–10 days with follow-up examination after the conclusion of treatment. A course

of treatment for 6 weeks followed by a 1-week taper may be necessary. The patient and family should be informed of the high potency of the steroid prescribed, and emphasis should be given to limit its time of use. The course of lichen sclerosus et atrophicus is variable, and parents (and, at an appropriate age, the patient) should be informed that this condition may be lifelong, or that it may wax and wane for many years.

Genital bleeding, especially when scant and associated with pruritus, may simply be related to excoriations from aggressive scratching. Scratching of the genital area, in particular in patients with longer fingernails, may lead to breaks in the skin that lead to bleeding. Causes of such pruritus may include pinworms, atopic dermatitis, contact dermatitis, tight undergarments, wet bathing suits, and insect bites. These causes are generally easily elucidated through the history and physical examination. In the case of pinworms, pruritis may be worst around the rectum and at night, and diagnosis may be made through tape-testing. Tape-testing can be performed by parents and involves a brief application of clear tape to the perirectal area while the child is sleeping at night. On inspection, one may directly visualize pinworms stuck to the tape. Pinworms are treated using oral anthelmintics, such as mebendazole. In addition, when a child is scratching the genitals so extensively that trauma occurs, trimming the fingernails is beneficial to minimize skin damage.

A final consideration in the young girl with vaginal bleeding, which will be discussed in detail in Chapter 3, is precocious puberty. Vaginal bleeding in response to estrogen exposure may be due to true precocious puberty or to an independent source of estrogen, such as exposure to exogenous estrogen in the form of oral contraceptive pills. Precocious puberty presents with not only vaginal bleeding, but also the other signs of pubertal development, including growth of the breasts and axillary and pubic hair, and a growth spurt with associated bone maturation. In this setting, the initial assessment should include a very careful history to search for exogenous hormonal exposure. Estrogen-producing ovarian or adrenal tumors generally present with rapid onset and progression of pubertal changes and can be detected by radiologic studies. McCune–

Albright syndrome is notable for irregular café-au-lait spots, polyostotic fibrous dysplasia, and gonadotropin releasing hormone-independent precocious puberty. Finally, the uncommon presentation of premature menarche is marked by single or periodic episodes of vaginal bleeding without other evidence of premature pubertal development. If the above causes are ruled out, an evaluation for true (or central) precocious puberty must be considered.

Malignant

Tumors of the vagina and cervix are rare in young girls. The most common form of soft tissue sarcoma in childhood is the rhabdomyosarcoma, of which approximately 20% involve the genitourinary tract. A subtype—sarcoma botryoides—is the most common malignant tumor of the genital tract of young girls, with a peak incidence occurring before 2 years of age. This almost always develops prior to age 5, with an average age at the time of diagnosis of 3 years. As a child's age increases, lesions tend to originate higher in the genital tract. The bimodal incidence of this cancer with a second peak of frequency in adolescence results in the manifestation of cervical tumors.

The characteristic description of presentation is passage of a polypoid, grape-like mass; however, more typical symptoms are vaginal bleeding or a bloody discharge. On examination, a soft, friable mass is present protruding from the vagina. Definitive diagnosis requires a biopsy of the lesion to distinguish it from the much rarer endodermal sinus tumor and other benign polypoid lesions, most typically condyloma acuminata. Sarcoma botryoides tends to arise in the anterior wall of the vagina, compared to endodermal sinus tumors, which originate in the posterior wall or vaginal fornices. The tumor is rapidly growing and very aggressive, requiring expert multimodality treatment. Contemporary therapeutic approaches endeavor to maintain normal anatomy and function and involve neoadjuvant multiagent chemotherapy followed by surgical excision of residual tumor. Radiation therapy is reserved for inadequate response to chemotherapy, treatment of remaining disease, or involvement of the lymph nodes. Survival rates are excellent at greater than 90% at 5 years.

> ### ♨ SCIENCE REVISITED
>
> Rhabdomyosarcoma is a malignant tumor of striated muscle origin. It is derived from primitive mesenchyme that retains its capacity for skeletal muscle differentiation. Of the five categories, embryonal rhabdomyosarcoma is the most common subtype, occurring in the walls of hollow, mucosa-lined structures such as the nasopharynx, common bile duct, urinary bladder, and vagina in females (i.e., head and neck and genitourinary systems). On histologic examination, they have high cytologic variability, which represents several stages of skeletal muscle morphogenesis. Embryonal rhabdomyosarcoma has unique molecular characteristics, showing a loss of specific genome material from the short arm of chromosome 11 (11p15 region), suggesting the presence of a tumor suppressor gene. Another molecular feature is its lack of gene amplification. In addition, the cellular DNA content is hyperdiploid (1.1–1.8 × normal DNA). The botryoid type, a subset of embryonal rhabdomyosarcoma, characteristically arises under the mucosal surfaces of body orifices, forming polypoid, grape-like tumor masses. On histologic study, botryoid rhabdomyosarcoma demonstrates malignant cells in an abundant myxoid stroma.

Genital tract endodermal sinus tumors are extremely rare, with only case reports in the literature. The presentation is similar to that of sarcoma botryoides, and these are the two important malignant neoplasms to consider in the diagnosis by biopsy.

Conclusions

Vaginal bleeding in prepubertal females can be distressing to young girls and their families; however, a thoughtful and careful history and physical examination will likely reveal a cause that is benign and readily treatable. A summary algorithm for the clinical approach to prepubertal genital bleeding is provided in Figure 2.6. Any concern for abuse, however, must be taken

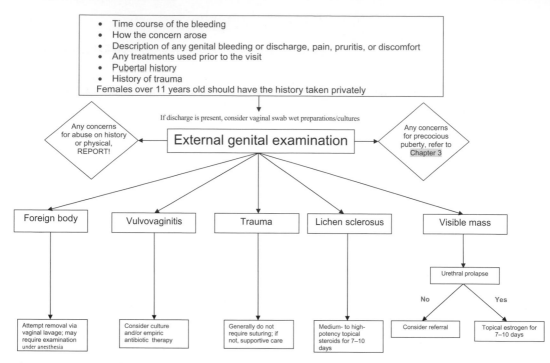

Figure 2.6 Approach to external genital examination.

seriously and reported to child protective services or law enforcement.

Selected bibliography

Berenson AB, Heger AH, Hayes JM, Bailey RK, Emans SJ. Appearance of the hymen in prepubertal girls. Pediatrics 1992;89:387–94.

Groff DB. Pelvic neoplasms in children. J Surg Oncol 2001;77:65–71.

Kass-Wolff JH. Pediatric gynecology: assessment strategies and common problems. Semin Reprod Med 2003;21:329–38.

Lara-Torre E. The physical examination in pediatric and adolescent patients. Clin Obstet Gynecol 2008;5100:205–13.

Maharaj NR, Nimako D, Hadley GP. Multimodal therapy for the initial management of genital embryonal rhabdomyosarcoma in childhood. Int J Gynecol Cancer 2008;18:190–2.

Sugar NF, Graham EA. Common gynecologic problems in prepubertal girls. Pediatr Rev 2006;27:213–23.

3

Irregular Vaginal Bleeding and Amenorrhea During the Pubertal Years

Bradley S. Hurst

Carolinas Medical Center, Charlotte, North Carolina, USA

Introduction

Puberty is a remarkable stage in life in which the adolescent matures from childhood to sexual maturity. Although the physiologic events are complex, in most circumstances the pubertal progression follows a predictable sequence within a fairly narrow interval, and in girls it is concluded when regular ovulatory menstrual cycles are established. However, this intricate system is susceptible to many types of error in maturation. Precocious pubertal development is a result of early exposure of sex steroids, either by activation of the hypothalamic–pituitary–ovarian (HPO) axis or by endogenous or exogenous exposure to reproductive hormones.

Delayed puberty occurs if there is failure to activate any component of the HPO axis.

Even if maturation of the HPO axis is normal, amenorrhea may indicate failure of the female reproductive tract to develop. Puberty is an especially turbulent phase, because almost all girls experience anovulatory bleeding during the first year after menarche. Because of the unpredictable nature of "normal" bleeding during puberty, it is a challenge to determine whether abnormal bleeding in an adolescent is temporary and expected to correct with maturation, or whether excessive bleeding indicates a more serious underlying disorder.

This chapter will focus on the challenges of evaluating and treating the adolescent with pubertal menstrual disorders by reviewing normal pubertal development, precious puberty, excessive bleeding during the pubertal years, delayed puberty, and amenorrhea.

⚛ SCIENCE REVISITED

Normal puberty follows a predictable sequence of development, although some variation is not unusual. During infancy and childhood, the hypothalamic secretion of gonadotropin-releasing hormone (GnRH) is suppressed by a central nervous control center termed the "gonadostat." During late childhood, there is an "awakening" of the hypothalamus, with secretion of pulsatile GnRH and luteinizing hormone, primarily at night. The cause of this awakening is not known, but it is partially related to increasing body mass and increasing levels of leptin, a hormone secreted by adipose tissue. Leptin receptors in the hypothalamus stimulate GnRH synthesis, and leptin-deficient girls fail to initiate puberty. As hypothalamic and pituitary maturation occurs, the pulse amplitude and frequency of luteinizing hormone and follicle-stimulating hormone increase. Eventually, gonadotropin levels stimulate the growth of an ovarian follicle, although the development of a mature follicle and ovulation do not occur until the

---

Disorders of Menstruation, 1st edition. Edited by Paul B. Marshburn and Bradley S. Hurst.

hypothalamic–pituitary–ovarian axis has matured. The developing follicle secretes estradiol, and low levels of estradiol initiate breast development.

Normal puberty, including irregular bleeding and dysmenorrhea

Breast development, known as thelarche, begins as the ovaries secrete estrogen in response to activation of the hypothalamic stimulation of pituitary gonadotropins. Thelarche is usually the first indication of puberty; it begins at 9–11 years of age and is completed in 3–3.5 years in most girls. Adrenarche, the development of sexual pubic and axillary hair, begins in response to an increase in adrenal androgens. Adrenarche is not strictly linked to thelarche, but usually begins soon after thelarche, typically between 11 and 12 years of age. Growth accelerates between ages 10 and 14, with peak growth at 12. Menarche, the first episode of vaginal bleeding, begins at approximately age 12.8, about 2.5 years after thelarche. Isolated menarche before age 10 is rare, and bleeding of this nature may indicate sexual abuse.

⚙ SCIENCE REVISITED

Pubertal development is abnormal when the timing of these events significantly deviates from normal, so it is important to consider normal variations. In the United States, 10% of girls begin thelarche by age 8, adrenarche by age 10, and menarche by age 11 years. Furthermore, there is considerable racial variation, so what is considered normal for one group may be atypical for another. For example, thelarche begins in 15% of African-American girls, but only 5% of white girls, by age 7. Thirty-five percent of African-American girls begin thelarche by age 8, compared to 10% of white girls. The onset of adrenarche is even more pronounced: at age 6, occurring in 10% of African-American girls and only 1% of white girls, with figures of 15% and 2% by age 7, 35% and 5% at age 8, and 60% and 20% by age 9.

Most vaginal bleeding that occurs in the first year after menarche is anovulatory. Anovulatory bleeding is characterized by irregular, unpredictable bleeding, in terms of timing, amount, and duration. In contrast, ovulatory cycles may be preceded by premenstrual symptoms such as bloating, breast soreness, or cramping. Dysmenorrhea, or menstrual-related cramping, usually indicates bleeding after an ovulatory cycle, although cramping occurs with the passage of uterine clots in both ovulatory and anovulatory cycles. Often, ovulatory and anovulatory cycles are interspersed until a regular ovulatory pattern is established.

Dysmenorrhea

Dysmenorrhea occurs in approximately two-thirds of teenage girls, with a peak incidence in the late teens and early 20s. Severe dysmenorrhea may be associated with nausea, vomiting, loose stools, or a combination of these, and pain may be so severe that absences from school are necessary. Usually, these symptoms are controlled with nonsteroidal anti-inflammatory drugs, especially ibuprofen or naproxen; many girls will experience the greatest symptomatic relief with the use of hormonal contraception: oral, vaginal, transdermal, or injectable. Continuous hormonal contraception is helpful for girls who experience severe dysmenorrhea associated with even slight bleeding.

If pain persists in spite of these measures, further evaluation should be initiated to assess for a uterine or vaginal obstruction. Magnetic resonance imaging (MRI) or laparoscopy is needed to evaluate for congenital anomalies that may cause obstruction and progressive pain in each cycle if the diagnosis is uncertain after physical and ultrasound examination. Obstructive abnormalities usually cause pain with the onset of the first menstrual period. Obstruction in the presence of menstruation may occur with an occluded hemivagina when there is cervical and uterine duplication from a didelphic, bicornuate, or septate uterus. Obstruction may also occur from an incompletely formed uterine horn with a functional endometrium and a contralateral normal unicornuate uterus (Figure 3.1). These obstructive conditions predispose to endometriosis by retrograde menstruation.

Endometriosis may provide an additional explanation for progressive dysmenorrhea, although typically the first menses are not painful. If ultrasound imaging is negative and endometriosis is suspected, laparoscopy may be needed to evaluate and treat endometriosis (see Chapter 9).

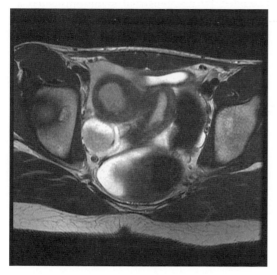

Figure 3.1 Magnetic resonance image of an obstructed incompletely formed uterine horn with a functional endometrium and a contralateral normal unicornuate uterus.

Precocious puberty—an evaluation algorithm (Figure 3.2)

Precocious puberty is a challenging topic for many gynecologists, especially since few gynecologists routinely see young adolescents and children. However, precocious pubertal development may be caused by serious underlying disorders. Furthermore, untreated precocious pubertal development may result in diminished height and result in psychological problems. Because of these important considerations, it is crucial that the girl with precocious puberty be evaluated and treated appropriately. An evaluation is considered appropriate for girls who begin to show signs of pubertal development before the age of 8 years.

Complete versus incomplete precocious puberty

It is important to define and differentiate types of precocious development into "complete" and "incomplete." "Complete" precocious puberty

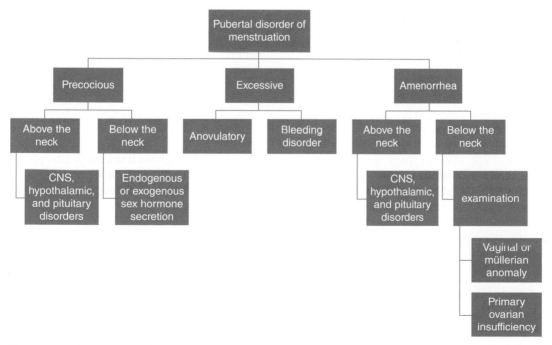

Figure 3.2 Algorithm for diagnosing precocious puberty. CNS, central nervous system

refers to the activation of the HPO axis that initiates pubertal development, whereas "incomplete" refers to sexual maturation caused primarily by hormone secretion or the presence of exogenous hormones. In general, complete precocity is caused by factors that occur "in the head" that cause activation of the HPO axis such as central nervous system (CNS) tumors, and incomplete precocity is caused by factors that originate below the neck, such as hormonally active ovarian tumors.

Isosexual versus heterosexual precious puberty

The terms "isosexual" and "heterosexual" are another important way to define precocious puberty. Isosexual precocious puberty follows the pattern of same sexual development; therefore, a girl feminizes. Heterosexual precocity follows the pattern of the opposite sex, meaning that a girl will masculinize. As might be expected, isosexual precocity is caused by secretion of estrogen, sometimes accompanied by progesterone, whereas heterosexual precocity is caused by androgens. Understanding these terms and their implications will help the physician limit the differential diagnosis and initiate the most appropriate diagnostic evaluation.

The differential diagnosis for precious puberty is long, and in order to simplify the evaluation it is worthwhile separating the underlying causes into two main categories: above (Table 3.1) and below the neck. Even with this approach, it is important to know that 75% of precocious puberty in girls is idiopathic, or unexplained. Potentially life-threatening causes may include CNS tumors, other serious CNS disorders, ovarian and adrenal tumors, and following treatment of congenital adrenal hyperplasia (CAH).

Complete precocious puberty

Complete precocious puberty occurs when pubertal development is initiated because of activation of the HPO axis. During late childhood, it becomes more likely that the etiology will be unexplained, whereas an organic cause is likely to trigger maturation in an infant or young child. Complete precocious puberty is caused by a loss of the inhibitory "gonadostat" that typically suppresses pulsatile gonadotropin-releasing hormone (GnRH) release from the hypothalamus, and therefore pulsatile follicle-stimulating hormone (FSH) and luteinizing hormone (LH) secretion from the pituitary; alternatively, stimulation of the HPO axis may be caused by an "irritating" factor such as a tumor. The result is an accelerated occurrence of pubertal development, manifested by early thelarche, adrenarche, the linear growth spurt, and menarche.

The physician must consider CNS tumors in the differential diagnosis of "above the neck" causes of precocious puberty (Table 3.1). These lesions can be identified by MRI of the pituitary with gadolinium contrast. Of the CNS tumors, the three most common are glioma, astrocytoma, and ependymoma. Craniopharyngioma is a common cause of delayed puberty and may cause secondary amenorrhea, but it rarely causes precocious puberty. A glioma is identified as a densely enhancing lesion near the optic chiasm. A hamartoma is not a true tumor but a complex

Table 3.1 Precocious puberty—10 "above the neck" causes

Central nervous system tumor: glioma, astrocytoma, ependyoma, craniopharyngioma (rare)
Hamartoma of the tuber cinereum
Hydrocephalus
Encephalitis
Brain abscess
Arachnoid cyst
Sarcoid granuloma
Tuberculous granuloma
Head trauma
Epilepsy

of neurosecretory neurons, fiber bundles, and glial cells. Hamartomas are a frequent cause of precocious puberty before age 3, and a child with a hamartoma often presents with seizures.

Other CNS causes of precocious puberty include physical conditions that affect the brain. The differential diagnosis includes hydrocephalus, encephalitis, brain abscess, and CNS granuloma. One key observation is the overall health of the child as these conditions are unlikely in a thriving child. Meningitis, seizures, and trauma may trigger precocious puberty, but these factors can often be elicited by the clinical history.

> ★ TIPS AND TRICKS
>
> Once maturation of the hypothalamic–pituitary–ovarian axis has occurred, pubertal development is likely to continue even after the initial problem has been resolved. Long-term administration of gonadotropin-releasing hormone (GnRH) agonists is needed to suppress the pituitary gonadotropins until the child reaches an age of normal puberty; at that time, GnRH agonist therapy may be discontinued to allow maturation to continue.

Incomplete isosexual precocious puberty

The differential diagnosis of incomplete (below the neck) precocious puberty (Table 3.2) is most conveniently separated into isosexual and heterosexual etiologies. Since incomplete precocious puberty implies a nonfunctional hypothalamic–pituitary–gonadal axis, the initiating etiology is caused by stimulation of pubertal development by sex steroids. Isosexual precocity implies exposure to estrogen and possibly progesterone, usually derived from the ovary or an extrinsic source, such as oral contraceptives (Table 3.2). Heterosexual precocity implies androgen stimulation, and this may originate from the ovary, the adrenal gland, or exogenous exposure (Table 3.3). Regardless of the initial source, exposure to sex steroids can cause maturation of the HPO axis, and puberty can advance even after the initial problem has been corrected.

Follicle cyst

Spontaneous growth and maturation of an ovarian follicle is the most common cause of isosexual precocity. Estradiol is produced as the follicle grows, and even a small rise in estrogen

Table 3.2 Incomplete isosexual precocious puberty—"below the neck" causes

Follicular cyst (most common)
Granulosa cell tumor (rare in childhood)
Theca cell tumor (third most common estrogen-secreting tumor)
McCune–Albright syndrome (polyostotic fibrous dysplasia)
Hypothyroid (expect failure to thrive)
Peutz–Jeghers syndrome (mucocutaneous pigmentation, gastrointestinal polyposis)
Exogenous hormones

Table 3.3 Incomplete heterosexual precocious puberty

Ovarian tumor
• Granulosa/theca cell • Sertoli–Leydig cells tumors (rare before the teens) • Dysgerminoma (*if* interstitial cells are present) • Gonadoblastoma (only XY pseudohermaphrodites)
Adrenal androgen tumor
Congenital adrenal hyperplasia
Exogenous androgens

levels can trigger thelarche. Symptom onset is rapid. In some cases, a simple ovarian follicle cyst can be demonstrated. However, a follicle cyst resolves rapidly without ovulation in girls with an immature HPO axis, and the decline in serum estrogen levels may initiate endometrial bleeding. There is often no evidence of a cyst by the time the child is brought in for medical evaluation. The condition is limited, and in the absence of estrogen some regression of thelarche may occur. However, girls who experience precocity due to a follicle cyst may have recurrent episodes.

The development of follicle cysts is explained by growth of a follicle in the absence of normal FSH and LH stimulation. During most of the prepubertal years, the hypothalamic secretion of GnRH is suppressed by the "gonadostat." However, throughout childhood, the ovaries contain follicles that begin to mature, but since the "gonadostat" inhibits FSH and LH pituitary secretion the follicles degenerate without making secreting appreciable levels of estradiol.

Ovarian neoplasm

A granulosa cell tumor of the ovary is a rare but serious cause of precocious puberty and is identified by the presence a solid or combined solid and cystic tumor in the ovary on ultrasound. Granulosa cell tumors are derived from the granulosa cells that surround the oocyte in an ovarian follicle. Just as granulosa cells secrete two primary measurable hormones, estradiol and inhibin, so granulosa cell tumors are identified by elevated levels of these two hormones. Because of the elevated estradiol levels, a granulosa cell tumor initiates isosexual puberty and stimulates breast development and accelerated growth.

Occasionally, a child presents with clitoromegaly and adrenarche caused by testosterone produced by the tumor. If the condition is untreated, uterine bleeding may occur by continuous estrogen stimulation of the endometrium or as estradiol levels decline if there is a fluctuation in estrogen levels. Eventually, chronic estrogen exposure may activate the HPO axis, so it may be necessary to treat with GnRH agonists after a granulosa cell tumor has been surgically removed. Granulosa cell tumors can be benign or malignant. In adults, they tend to be slow growing and may recur many years after surgical removal, but recurrence in children often occurs before 3 years has passed. Overall, 20% die of recurrent disease.

Theca cell tumors are the third most common estrogen-secreting tumor. These tumors are derived from the theca cells that surround the granulosa cells in an ovarian follicle. The theca cells can produce androgens, estrogens, and, if luteinized, progesterone. A granulosa–theca cell tumor has components of granulosa and theca cells. As might be predicted, theca cell tumors may stimulate concurrent isosexual and heterosexual development. Theca cell tumors have a solid or combined solid and cystic appearance on ultrasound. Management is the same as for granulosa cell tumors—primarily surgical removal—but these are usually benign. Estradiol and inhibin are less useful markers for these neoplasms.

McCune–Albright syndrome

McCune–Albright syndrome, also referred to as polyostotic fibrous dysplasia, causes isosexual precocious puberty due to ovarian secretion of estradiol as a result of a congenital G protein abnormality (see "Science revisited" below). The syndrome is diagnosed when at least two of the following features are found: (1) irregular cutaneous café-au-lait spots; (2) polyostotic fibrous dysplasia; and (3) sexual precocity due to autonomous hyperfunction. The café-au-lait spots have jagged borders like the coast of Maine, and rarely cross the midline. The bone defects affect the long bones in the arms and legs, pelvis, ribs, skull, and facial bones. Less commonly, the spine and clavicle may be affected. These defects may cause fractures and deformities.

McCune–Albright syndrome is caused by a postnatal mosaic defect in the gene that codes for the guanine nucleotide-binding protein, alpha-stimulating activity polypeptide (*GNAS*); varying degrees of severity may be found. The defect in the *GNSA1* gene results in continuous stimulation of adenyl cyclase and elevated cyclic adenosine monophosphate levels.

Treatment of McCune–Albright syndrome is directed at suppressing estradiol production. In the past, testolactone and ketoconazole were utilized, but the aromatase inhibitors including letrozole and anastrazole may now be preferred due to fewer side effects. Inhibition of the enzyme aromatase blocks the production of estradiol from testosterone and slows pubertal progression. As precocity is caused by autonomous stimulation of ovarian estradiol, GnRH agonists are ineffective as primary treatment, although they may be useful to suppress FSH and LH if maturation of the HPO axis has occurred. Interestingly, reproductive function with McCune–Albright syndrome is normal as an adult.

Peutz–Jeghers syndrome, also known as hereditary intestinal polyposis syndrome, is an autosomal dominant condition characterized by benign hamartomatous polyps in the gastrointestinal tract, dark pigmented macules in the mouth, eyes, nostrils, lips, and anus, and sometimes an associated precocious puberty. Peutz–Jeghers syndrome is caused by a mutation in the *STK11* gene and has an estimated incidence of one in 300,000. Affected individuals may present with an intussusceptions or bowel obstruction. The cause of precocious puberty in these individuals is sex cord tumors of the ovary.

Profound hypothyroidism is a rare cause of precocious puberty in developed countries, primarily because most severe cases of severe hypothyroidism are diagnosed and treated. Affected children fail to grow adequately, and their physical and verbal development lags far behind expected norms. Arrhythmias may occur. Correction of the condition with thyroid replacement is the primary treatment.

Exogenous hormones

Exogenous hormonal exposure should be considered in all cases of sexual precocity, and consideration for this diagnosis is heightened when the initial evaluation fails to identify an underlying cause. It may be difficult to identify the source of estrogen or progesterone exposure, and the family should be carefully questioned for use of hormonal contraception with birth control pills, patches, or the vaginal ring. The use of transdermal estrogen therapy is becoming increasingly popular for symptomatic menopausal women, and a child may show signs of pubertal development with even low levels of exposure. Estrogenic substances in the environment have been suggested as a possible but still unproven cause of precocious puberty.

Heterosexual precocious puberty

Heterosexual precocious puberty is caused by exposure to androgens, with masculine pattern pubertal development dominated by adrenarche and, when severe, virilizing development that may include clitoromegaly and terminal hair growth on the chest, upper abdomen, face, neck, and back. Heterosexual precocious puberty accelerates linear growth, but early fusion of the epiphyseal plates subsequently results in short stature. The masculine pubertal development causes profound social stigma, and psychological stress occurs in many girls. Virilizing changes tend to be irreversible, so immediate attention is required to identify and treat the underlying cause. The most common causes of heterosexual precocious puberty include ovarian androgen-secreting tumors and CAH.

Sex cord stromal tumors are derived from the hormonally active cells in the ovary. These tumors can secrete androgens, and if they are active during childhood, androgen-secreting tumors cause heterosexual precocious puberty. Granulosa and/or theca cell tumors, discussed above, primarily secrete estrogens but will cause masculinization if appreciable levels of testosterone are produced. Sertoli–Leydig tumors are rare before the teen years and are therefore a rare cause of precocity. A dysgerminoma can be hormonally active, but only if interstitial cells are present. Gonadoblastomas are found in XY pseudohermaphrodites.

Congenital adrenal hyperplasia

CAH causes heterosexual precocious puberty when corticosteroid replacement is insufficient to suppress adrenocorticotropin (ACTH) levels. Elevated ACTH levels increase the initiation of adrenal steroidogenesis, and androgen production and secretion increases and stimulates masculine pubertal development: adrenarche, mature body odor, and a linear growth spurt. The extent of masculinization depends on the severity of the enzyme defect and the degree of undertreatment. Adequate adrenal suppression is assessed with 17-hydroxyprogesterone (17-OHP) and testosterone levels. These children should be assessed by charting growth rates, with determination of bone age every year or two. If the HPO axis has been activated by the elevated androgens, prolonged GnRH agonist therapy should be initiated and continued until the normal age of puberty. Aromatase inhibitors such as testolactone or letrozole and antiandrogens such as flutamide may reduce the masculinizing consequences of CAH and reduce the risk of short stature due to premature epiphyseal closure.

⚗ SCIENCE REVISITED

Congenital adrenal hyperplasia (CAH) is caused by autosomal recessive abnormalities in genes that code for enzymes involved in the synthesis of adrenal cortisol from cholesterol. Several enzymatic defects can cause CAH: 21-hydroxylase deficiency, responsible for over 95% of cases, 3-beta-hydroxysteroid dehydrogenase deficiency, and 11-beta-hydroxylase deficiency, which also cause hypertension. Normally, cortisol production in the adrenal gland is stimulated by pituitary adrenocorticotropin (ACTH), but in CAH cortisol production is partially or completely blocked by the enzymatic defect. Adrenal androgen secretion increases as these intermediate precursors to cortisol accumulate. Low cortisol levels cause an increase in ACTH, which further stimulates androgen production. CAH is a common cause of ambiguous genitalia, since androgen levels increase in utero. Depending on the severity of the gene defect, salt-wasting 21-hydroxylase CAH can cause ambiguous genitalia due to insufficient cortisol and aldosterone production, simple virilizing CAH causes ambiguous genitalia and precocious puberty, and late-onset adrenal hyperplasia can cause ovulatory dysfunction and infertility. Newborn screening programs detect CAH at birth, and infants are treated with glucocorticoid and mineralocorticoid replacement.

Adrenal androgen-secreting tumor

Adenomas of the adrenal cortex are benign tumors, approximately 15% secreting steroid hormones, including androgen, corticosteroids (Cushing syndrome), or mineralocorticoids (Conn syndrome). Most are less than 2 cm in size. They can cause ovulatory dysfunction and virilization in women, but are very uncommon in young women and a rare cause of precocious puberty.

Adrenocortical carcinoma is a rare cancer of adrenal cortical cells and may occur in children. Some secrete androgens, and heterosexual pubertal development may be one of the first indicators of this aggressive cancer. Most often, these tumors are large when initially diagnosed.

Exogenous androgens

Just as exogenous estrogen exposure can initiate isosexual precocious puberty, exposure to androgens can initiate heterosexual pubertal development in girls. Although androgen exposure has been an uncommon occurrence in the past, testosterone gels and patches are increasingly prescribed to improve wellbeing in both men and women, and are used illicitly by some athletes and body-builders. An increasing availability raises the risk of exposure during the prepubertal years. The availability of any androgenic substance must be determined by carefully questioning family members any time a girl presents with heterosexual precocity.

Evaluation of isosexual precocious puberty—an algorithm (Table 3.4)

In order for the clinician to perform a meaningful evaluation of a girl with isosexual precocious

Table 3.4 Evaluation of precocious puberty

History
• Age of onset, growth, exogenous hormone exposure

Examination
• Growth curves
• Tanner stage
• Genital examination
• Secondary sexual development
• Neurologic examination
• Visual field examination
• Optic discs
• Skin lesions
• Abdominal and pelvic masses

Radiologic studies
• Bone age
• Magnetic resonance imaging/computed tomography of the head
• Pelvic ultrasound

Laboratory studies
• Luteinizing hormone, follicle-stimulating hormone, estradiol
• Gonadotropin-releasing hormone stimulation test
• Thyroid function tests

Heterosexual puberty: add 17-hydroxyprogesterone, dehydroepiandrosterone sulfate, testosterone, ±24-hour urinary cortisol

puberty, it is most important to understand the components of the differential diagnosis. For that reason, the differential diagnosis is considered when initiating the evaluation. The key aspects of the evaluation are to identify life-threatening conditions, to correct underlying causes of precocious development, and to prevent further development. Simultaneously, the clinician must be aware of the psychological state of the patient, her family, and friends, and counseling should be strongly encouraged.

History

The time of onset of breast development, sexual hair, growth, and adult body odor should be elicited by the history. Conditions that affect the general wellbeing should be explored, and in children this includes the achievement of developmental milestones and performance in school. Chronic illnesses and failure to grow and thrive may indicate more serious underlying health conditions. Although it may be difficult to elicit specific complaints, a behavioral history should include questions about the child's level of irritability and aggressive behavior. Headaches, nausea, vomiting, visual difficulties, or seizures may indicate a CNS-related condition but could also indicate an intra-abdominal problem. Evaluation of growth curves can help the provider to identify the onset of an underlying cause of precocious development. A history of severe head trauma should be assessed. The provider should determine if there is a family history of precocious puberty, and if there are any hormone-containing medications or products in the home or at the homes of friends and family members.

Examination

A comprehensive examination should be performed, with special attention to assessment of Tanner stage (Figure 3.3), genital examination, and examination of secondary sexual development. However, a measurement of the breast tissue at right angles, horizontally, and vertically

(a)

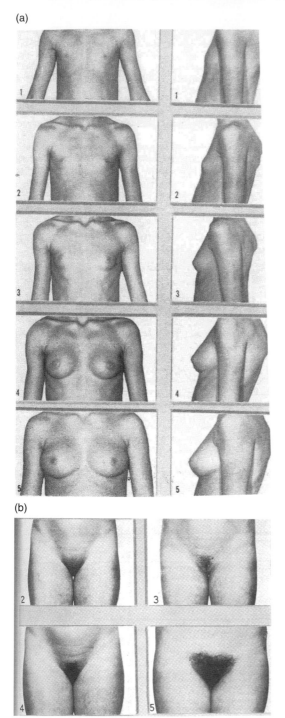

(b)

Figure 3.3 Tanner stage breast and pubic hair. Breast: Tanner I, prepubertal; II, breast bud; III, breast extends beyond areolar borders; IV, areola forms secondary mound; V, adult. Pubic hair: Tanner I, prepubertal; II, long soft hair on labia majora; III, coarse, curly hair; IV, extends across pubis but not medial thighs; V, adult hair to medial thigh.

◄───────────────────────────

allows for a more reproducible assessment of development than Tanner staging. Breast tissue is firm, sub- and periareolar, and distinctly different from the soft surrounding fat tissue. A change in nipple color from light pink to brown suggests exposure to progesterone, a product of ovulation or exogenous hormones. A neurologic examination should be done, and visual fields and optic discs assessed, if the patient is cooperative. A careful examination of skin lesions, especially café-au-lait blotches or mucocutaneous pigmentation, may suggest McCune–Albright syndrome or Peutz–Jeghers syndrome. Abdominal masses should be assessed by abdominal examination, and pelvic masses should be assessed by rectal examination, if the patient is cooperative.

Radiologic studies

An MRI with gadolinium contrast pituitary will identify most CNS lesions that cause precocious puberty, although a calcified craniopharyngioma is most readily identified by computed tomography (CT) imaging. A pelvic and abdominal ultrasound will identify most ovarian tumors or identify a follicle cyst, if present (Figure 3.4). Ultrasound can also be used to determine the endometrial thickness, an indirect assessment of the current estrogen status, as discussed in other chapters. Bone age can be determined by the use of special wrist film, with Bayley–Pinneau tables to determine whether bone age is advanced, and predicted height can be assessed.

Laboratory studies

LH, FSH, and estradiol levels are recommended for evaluation of isosexual precocious puberty. With a resolved follicle cyst, all of these will be low. The estradiol level is elevated if a functional follicle or estrogen-secreting tumor is present.

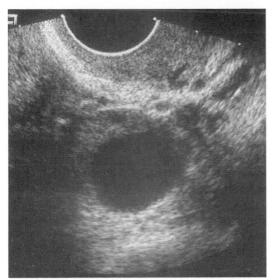

Figure 3.4 Ultrasound image of a follicle cyst.

Serum estradiol levels considered low in the adult woman (≤30 pg/mL) may cause rapid growth and premature closure of long bone epiphyses, with resulting short adult stature. If ultrasound imaging of the pelvis indicates the presence of a solid or solid and cystic mass, an inhibin level should be obtained as a preoperative marker of a granulosa cell tumor. Thyroid function tests, thyroid-stimulating hormone, and free thyroxine levels will screen for hypothyroidism.

Evaluation of heterosexual precocious puberty

> ⚙ **SCIENCE REVISITED**
>
> A gonadotropin-releasing hormone (GnRH) stimulation test is recommended to determine if there has been maturation of the hypothalamic–pituitary–ovarian axis. GnRH 100 μg is given as an intravenous bolus, and luteinizing hormone and follicle-stimulating hormone levels are obtained at 30 minutes. A minimal increase indicates an immature hypothalamic–pituitary axis. A twofold increase indicates activation, and in this case suppression with GnRH analogs is recommended until the child reaches the normal age of puberty, in order to delay puberty and maximize growth potential.

The evaluation is similar for the evaluation of heterosexual precocious puberty, except that the history and physical examination are targeted towards the differential diagnosis, primarily ovarian, adrenal, and exogenous sources of androgen exposure. Onset of adrenarche and course of progression, growth acceleration, onset of adult body odor, and presence or absence of breast development are key aspects of the history. Growth curves should be examined, evidence of pain, failure to thrive, abdominal distention, potential androgen availability in the home or with friends or family, history of adrenal hyperplasia, and assessment of compliance with treatment are examples of a focused history based on the differential diagnosis.

Physical examination

Although it is essential to perform a comprehensive physical examination, a focused examination should be performed considering the differential diagnosis. Therefore, the provider must assess androgenic signs including the extent of sexual hair, genital virilization, acne, breast development, Cushingoid signs such as truncal obesity and peripheral wasting, and abdominal palpation for masses. If tolerated, a rectal examination can determine whether a pelvic (ovarian) mass is present.

Laboratory studies

Laboratory studies include 17-OHP, dehydroepiandrosterone sulfate (DHEAS), testosterone, and possibly a 24-hour urine free cortisol collection. The 17-OHP level is elevated in 21-hydroxylase deficiency adrenal hyperplasia or when treatment of CAH is inadequate. DHEAS is secreted by the adrenal gland, and a marked elevation raises the suspicion of an adrenal androgen-producing tumor. Testosterone is secreted by the adrenal glands and ovaries, and a marked elevation raises the suspicion of either an ovarian or an adrenal androgen-secreting tumor. A 24-hour urine cortisol level is obtained if the patient has manifestations of Cushing syndrome. Further testing with low- and high-dose dexamethasone suppression tests is necessary to confirm the diagnosis of Cushing syndrome.

Pelvic ultrasound and adrenal computed tomography imaging

Unless a clear etiology is identified to explain the heterosexual development, such as incompletely treated CAH or obvious exogenous androgen exposure, an abdominal pelvic ultrasound should be obtained, and if an ovarian mass is not identified, adrenal CT imaging should be carried. However, an abdominal CT should be ordered before ultrasound if an adrenal tumor is suspected from an elevated DHEAS level or suspicion of Cushing syndrome.

Psychosocial implications of precocity

Early pubertal development may increase teasing and may result in later body image dissatisfaction. Precocious development increases the risk for physical sexual abuse. Precocious development sometimes unfairly raises expectations in adults that the child should be expected to achieve a higher level of performance in school and sports, and be more mature. Ongoing counseling should be encouraged to help the patient and family cope with these complex issues.

Excessive bleeding

Excessive bleeding is a common occurrence during puberty. Most often, heavy menses is the result of anovulatory bleeding, either related to irregular and prolonged cycles as the HPO axis matures, or the result of hyperandrogenism. Other serious causes must be considered for the adolescent with excessive bleeding, including neoplasms, pregnancy, trauma, physical abuse, and bleeding disorders.

Irregular, anovulatory cycles are most common at the beginning and the end of the reproductive years. In the adolescent, periods may be anovulatory for a year or more after menarche. Before the HPO axis is fully functional, FSH and LH secretion allows growth of a follicle, and estradiol is secreted. Estradiol stimulates endometrial proliferation, and the endometrium may continue to thicken until ovulation occurs, when the endometrium matures and then uniformly sheds with menses approximately 2 weeks after ovulation. A prolonged interval from menses to ovulation results in excessive ovulatory menstrual bleeding. Furthermore, if ovulation does not occur, the endometrium proliferates until irregular, unpredictable, sometimes heavy bleeding occurs. Eventually, regular ovulatory cycles are established for most adolescents. However, this irregular pattern is likely to continue in a teenager with polycystic ovarian syndrome (see Chapter 5).

Neoplasia is an unlikely cause of excessive genital bleeding in adolescents. Sarcoma botryoides usually occurs in young children, but cases have been reported after childhood. Other endometrial, cervical, and vaginal cancers are rare. However, genital condylomas or cervicitis may be identified in a sexually active or physically abused adolescent, so the physician must consider these in the differential diagnosis. A complete examination should help to raise or lower the suspicion of these diagnoses.

✋ CAUTION!

Pregnancy and pregnancy-related complications may be the cause of excessive bleeding. The fear of repercussions for admitting that a teenager has had intercourse, either consensual or the result of abuse, will cause many girls to deny that they could be pregnant. As many of the causes of bleeding during pregnancy can be life-threatening, a pregnancy test should always be performed, even if the likelihood of pregnancy appears to be minimal. If the pregnancy test is positive, the differential diagnosis for bleeding includes all the causes of pregnancy-related bleeding. Therefore, first-trimester bleeding may be caused by a threatened abortion (bleeding in pregnancy), missed abortion (fetal demise but no passage of tissue), incomplete abortion (passage of fetal tissue but the cervix is still open), ectopic pregnancy, complications of a pregnancy termination (legal or illegal), or bleeding from gestational trophoblastic disease (a molar pregnancy). In the second or third trimester, bleeding may indicate placental abruption or a placenta previa. All of these conditions are ruled out by a negative serum pregnancy test.

Table 3.5 Disorders of coagulation

Von Willebrand disease
Vitamin K deficiency (nutritional deficiency is rare)
Warfarin ingestion (medical treatment or accidental ingestion of rat poison)
Heparin or low molecular weight heparin administration
Disseminated intravascular coagulation (sepsis, trauma, obstetric, cancer)
Hemophilia (recessive, X-chromosome linked; rare in girls)
Aspirin
Thrombocytopenia
• Decreased production (such as vitamin B_{12} or folic acid deficiency, leukemia, sepsis) • Increased destruction (such as idiopathic thrombocytopenic purpura, thrombotic thrombocytopenic purpura, hemolytic–uremic syndrome, hypersplenism with splenic destruction of platelets, human immunodeficiency virus) • Medication-induced (such as chemotherapeutic agents, H2 receptor blockers, proton pump inhibitors) • Immunologic platelet destruction (such as quinidine)
Liver failure
Uremia
Congenital afibrinogenemia
Factor V deficiency
Factor X deficiency
Factor II deficiency (prothrombin deficiency)
Glanzmann's thrombasthenia (rare)
Bernard–Soulier syndrome (rare)

Bleeding disorders

Bleeding disorders are responsible for approximately 5–20% of hospital admissions for adolescents with excessive bleeding. Heavy periods may be the first indicator of coagulation disorders. Any factor that prevents the normal coagulation process during menstrual bleeding may be responsible. This can include disorders of platelets, von Willebrand disease, and clotting factor deficiencies. Platelet disorders that should be considered in adolescents include idiopathic thrombocytopenic purpura, leukemia, and hypersplenism. Other conditions related to excessive bleeding include vitamin K deficiency and aspirin or other medications that affect clotting (Table 3.5).

Von Willebrand disease

Von Willebrand disease is the most common inherited coagulation disorder that causes excessive bleeding, present in approximately 1 in 100 individuals, although it is clinically apparent in approximately 1 in 10,000. Von Willebrand disease may also be acquired in patients with autoantibodies. Von Willebrand disease is caused by a deficiency of the von Willebrand factor (vWF), a protein responsible for platelet adhesion. Although von Willebrand disease may first be suspected due to heavy menses, other signs and symptoms include easy bruising, nosebleeds, and excessive bleeding with trauma or surgery.

> **⚙ SCIENCE REVISITED**
>
> There are multiple types of von Willebrand disease, and the various presentations make this a confusing diagnostic problem for many providers. Type 1, responsible for 60–80% of all von Willebrand disease, is an autosomal

dominant deficiency of von Willebrand factor (vWF), usually being 10–40% of normal. Most individuals with type 1 disease live normal lives but may experience heavy periods, excessive bleeding with surgery, trauma, or dental extractions, and easy bruising. Type 2 is responsible for 20–30% of the cases, and is usually caused by an autosomal dominant defect in the vWF protein. The severity of the disease is related to the functional capacity of the faulty protein. In assays, the vWF levels are normal, but vWF activity is low. There are four subtypes: 2A, 2B, 2M, and 2N. In subtype 2B, the vWF spontaneously binds to platelets and causes a rapid clearance of platelets; a mild thrombocytopenia may occur. Because of increased platelet aggregation with this subtype, desmopressin should not be used to treat bleeding. Type 3 is the most severe form of the disease, with a bleeding pattern similar to that seen with hemophilia. Type 3 is caused by a homozygous defect in which there may be no detectable vWF antigen.

Evaluation and treatment of severe menorrhagia

Concurrent evaluation and treatment may be required when bleeding is life-threatening. A structured history and examination with the focus on the differential diagnosis should help to narrow the possible causes. A family history of bleeding disorders may raise the suspicion of von Willebrand disease. In addition to a complete general examination and pelvic examination, evidence of petechiae may indicate a bleeding disorder. An abnormal neurologic examination may be found with hemolytic–uremic syndrome.

If bleeding is severe, a large-bore intravenous catheter should be placed and fluid resuscitation initiated immediately while laboratory studies are obtained. Transfusions of packed red cells may be needed to maintain a satisfactory hemodynamic state. Ultrasound examination provides information on the possible cause of bleeding. In addition, ultrasound gives insight into the state of the ovaries, such as the presence of an ovarian follicle, and the endometrial thickness. A denuded endometrium is thin and is likely to respond best

to estrogen, and dysfunctional bleeding from a thick endometrium may respond best to progestin therapy or combined oral contraceptives.

★ TIPS & TRICKS

The initial laboratory studies should include a complete blood count and a serum pregnancy test. If a coagulation disorder is suspected, additional tests should be drawn: prothrombin time, activated partial thromboplastin time (if this is prolonged, obtain a mixing assay with pooled normal plasma to evaluate for inhibitor or factor deficiency), vonWillebrand factor (vWF) antigen, ristocetin cofactor, factor VIII, ABO type, Ivy bleeding time and/or Platelet Function Analyzer-100 closure time. If vWF levels are reduced, a thyroid-stimulating hormone level should be obtained, and a baseline iron profile should be obtained before administering a blood transfusion. If all of these studies are normal, consider platelet aggregation and release studies. If all studies are normal, consider factors XI and XII, euglobuin clot lysis studies, and other measures of fibrinolysis including alpha-2 antiplasmin levels, and plasminogen activator inhibitor level. These studies should be obtained with concurrent consultation with a hematologist. Consultation is especially valuable considering that vWF and factor VIII levels can fluctuate due to endogenous and exogenous hormonal factors.

Treatment of severe menorrhagia in adolescents

Acute profuse bleeding may be treated with one of two regimens: conjugated equine estrogen 2.5 mg or oral contraceptives four times daily. Ideally, the choice would be based on the endometrial pattern seen with ultrasound: a thin endometrium should be responsive to estrogen to induce proliferation and healing of a denuded cavity, whereas a thick endometrium should respond best to oral contraceptive therapy. The progestin allows for maturation of the endometrium and eventually an organized withdrawal bleeding at a later time.

When bleeding is life-threatening, oral contraceptives administered four times daily or intravenous conjugated equine estrogen 25 mg is given every 4 hours up to 24 hours, until bleeding has been controlled. The treatment is best determined by the endometrial thickness, with oral contraceptives being used when the endometrium is thick. Over 90% of individuals respond to treatment, but nausea and vomiting may be severe. If bleeding continues to be severe after one or two doses in spite of these measures, a hysteroscopy should be performed to evaluate the bleeding and, if possible, focal bleeding sites coagulated.

After the bleeding has been controlled, it is important to prevent recurrent episodes of anovulatory bleeding. In adolescents, this can be accomplished with cyclic progestin or hormonal contraception.

Physiologic delay of puberty

Evaluation of delayed puberty

An evaluation is warranted when a girl fails to achieve normal pubertal milestones within typical ages. The age of puberty varies bases on country and ethnic group. In the United States, 97% of girls have initiated thelarche by age 13, and other pubertal milestones occur over a period of 3–5 years. The absence of breast development by 13, menarche by 16, or an arrest of development may be due to a "constitutional delay." Delayed pubertal development may be dismissed by the patient and her parents, especially if the delay follows a familial pattern or is attributed to athletics or a small body frame. However, serious underlying causes should be ruled out by an evaluation.

Primary amenorrhea—an algorithm

Delayed puberty and primary amenorrhea can be divided into "above the neck" and below the neck" causes just as was done for precocious puberty, but congenital abnormalities of the reproductive tract must also be considered. "Above the neck" causes include still poorly defined stressors of the CNS that override and suppress hypothalamic functioning, including anorexia, low body weight, extreme physical exertion, starvation, and stress. Tumors of the CNS, hypothalamus or pituitary, or congenital defects of the HPO axis, can cause pubertal delay and primary amenorrhea. Ovarian disorders, primarily ovarian failure, is the most common cause of "below the neck" causes. Finally, there is a "below the waist" category for primary amenorrhea, due to müllerian anomalies, that is typically associated with normal thelarche but primary amenorrhea. Understanding the differential diagnosis is essential to performing the most efficient evaluation.

CNS amenorrhea and pubertal delay

Several CNS factors can cause pubertal delay and primary or secondary amenorrhea. Depending on the onset of the underlying problem, pubertal development is prevented if the onset of the underlying disorder occurs early. Puberty begins and then stops if the problem arises during puberty. Several CNS tumors cause delayed puberty.

A craniopharyngioma is the most common tumor causing delay. This tumor has a peak incidence between 6 and 14 years of age. It is usually suprasellar, arising in Rathke's pouch. Given the location, the most common signs and symptoms include visual defects, optic atrophy, or papilledema. As these tumors affect pituitary function, it is common to have an associated reduction in growth hormone and slowed growth, reduced thyroid function, and reduced ACTH and cortisol; diabetes insipidus may occur. Approximately 70% of these tumors are calcified.

Germinomas are the most common extrasellar tumor causing pubertal delay. The peak incidence occurs between 10 and 20 years of age. Presenting signs and symptoms commonly include diabetes insipidus and growth hormone deficiency. Visual changes are common. These tumors may secrete human chorionic gonadotropin, and if so, this can be a marker for clinical response to treatment. Germinomas are highly radiosensitive.

Other tumors and CNS abnormalities are less common but should be considered in certain clinical contexts. For example, the incidence of gliomas and astrocytomas is increased with neurofibromatosis. Histocyte disorders, including Hand–Schüller–Christian Disease, are associated with diabetes insipidus, growth hormone deficiency, bone cysts, and floating teeth. Midline teratomas and endodermal sinus tumors are rare causes of pubertal delay. Inflammatory conditions such as tuberculosis and sarcoid granuloma are rare cause of amenorrhea. Metastatic tumors, severe head trauma, and irradiation can also cause primary amenorrhea and pubertal delay.

Hypothalamic and pituitary-related pubertal delay

Prolactinomas comprise 40% of pituitary adenomas. Prolactinomas are uncommon in children and are more likely to cause a slowing or cessation of pubertal development instead of preventing the initiation of puberty. Pituitary prolactinomas are suspected when repeated prolactin levels are elevated, and a pituitary adenoma is confirmed with MRI. However, a large mass and prolactin levels less than 200 ng/mL should prompt the provider to look for excessive levels of other pituitary hormones including growth hormone and ACTH, and to consider a pituitary glycoprotein-secreting tumor.

Management of pituitary adenomas depends on their size and symptoms. Most pituitary microadenomas do not progress, and therefore expectant management is appropriate, with monitoring of symptoms, intermittent prolactin levels, and intermittent pituitary imaging (Figure 3.5). When indicated, medical treatment with bromocriptine or cabergoline (Dostinex) results

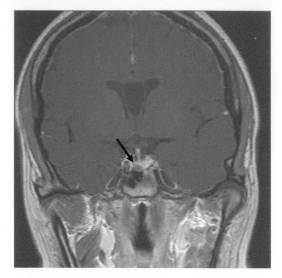

Figure 3.5 Pituitary magnetic resonance image showing a microadenoma (arrow).

in a decrease to normal prolactin levels in two-thirds of individuals with micro- or macroadenomas. Approximately 50% achieve a reduction in tumor size by 50% or more, and menses are restored in 80% with secondary amenorrhea, with a mean time of 5–6 weeks. If treatment is stopped, 40% experience recurrent amenorrhea within 4–5 weeks. Surgery is reserved for unresponsive tumors, but the recurrence rate after surgery is 30% for microadenomas and 90% for macroadenomas.

Congenital hypothalamic anomalies

Congenital anomalies can result in the absence of pubertal development and amenorrhea by causing a state of hypogonadotropic hypogonadism, or absent gonadal function due to insufficient secretion of hypothalamic GnRH.

Kallman syndrome
Kallman syndrome is caused by a congenital failure of the GnRH neurons to migrate from the olfactory placode to the hypothalamus during fetal development. The olfactory bulbs also fail to form, and individuals with Kallman syndrome have anosmia or hyposmia. In girls, Kallman syndrome is inherited as an autosomal dominant or recessive trait, but is also an X-linked recessive condition in males.

Individuals with Kallman syndrome ovulate with pulsatile GnRH pump or with gonado-tropin ovulation induction, so girls and their families should be counseled that the prognosis for future pregnancy is excellent. In order to achieve optimal pubertal breast development, it is recommended to use low-dose estrogen such as conjugated equine estrogen 0.3 mg daily for 6–12 months, with intermittent progestin withdrawal initially, since the use of oral contraceptives may lead to the development of "tubular" breasts. After breast development is satisfactory, low-dose hormone therapy or oral contraceptives may be used to maximize bone mineralization and complete pubertal development.

Other congenital syndromes with hypothalamic dysfunction

Prader–Willi syndrome is caused by gene dele-tions or unexpressed genes on the long arm of the paternally contributed chromosome 15. Maternal genes are silenced by imprinting. The condition is associated with hypogonadism, hypomenta-tion, hypotonia, and obesity. The incidence occurs in approximately 1 in 25,000 newborns. Bardet–Biedl syndrome is characterized by poly-dactyly, obesity, mental retardation, retinitis pig-mentosa, and hypogonadism.

"Below the neck" causes of delayed puberty or amenorrhea: primary ovarian insufficiency

Primary ovarian insufficiency, formerly referred to as "premature ovarian failure" or "premature menopause," is the preferred term used to describe early depletion of follicles from the ovaries of young women, or "hypergonadotropic hypogonadism." The laboratory hallmark is an elevated FSH level and a low estradiol level. In adolescents, primary ovarian insufficiency may be caused by serious underlying medical disor-ders, and has potential lifelong implications for health and fertility. The most common causes in adolescents include idiopathic, autoimmune, Turner syndrome, and the fragile X per-mutation. Other conditions include syndromes of gonadal dysgenesis, accelerated destruction of oocytes by chemotherapy or radiation therapy, and rare genetic disorders such as galactosemia.

Turner syndrome

Turner syndrome occurs in approximately 1 in 2,700 liveborn females and occurs when the second X chromosome is absent. Mosaic forms of Turner syndrome occurs due to postmeiotic errors, and the presentation may be more subtle than 45,X Turner syndrome. The monosomy X karyotype is the most common chromosome anomaly in spontaneous abortions. Less than 3% of 45,X fetuses survive to term.

Physical manifestations of Turner syndrome include short stature in 100% of those with monosomy X and 80% of those with Turner mosaicism. The incidence of streak gonads is 90% in both cases, and shield chest occurs in 75–80% in both forms. Other manifestations that are more common in the 45,X Turner syndrome than the mosaic form include hypoplastic nails, short forth metacarpal, webbed neck, multiple nevi, and lymphedema.

Loss of an X chromosome accelerates oocyte depletion. Although streak gonads are most common, approximately 8% of girls with mono-somy X Turner syndrome, and approximately 20% of those with Turner mosaicism, undergo menarche. Thus, it is not uncommon for a girl with Turner syndrome to begin pubertal develop-ment but then experience arrested maturation.

The presentation of Turner syndrome is similar or identical to another syndrome of gonadal dysgenesis—46,XY Swyer syndrome. Girls with Swyer syndrome are predisposed to gonadal cancer, so gonadectomy is indicated when a 46,XY karyotype is identified.

⚠ CAUTION

Although oocyte donation was considered an option for pregnancy in the past, Turner syndrome is now considered to be a relative contraindication to pregnancy, and Turner syndrome with coexistent cardiac disease is an absolute contraindication to pregnancy. Compared to an individual with a normal karyotype, a woman with Turner syndrome has a 100-fold increased risk of death with pregnancy, i.e., approximately 2% overall.

Pubertal development is promoted with low-dose estrogen, such as conjugated equine estrogen 0.3 mg daily or an estrogen patch 0.0375 mg with intermittent progestin therapy initially to promote more normal breast development and avoid the "tubular breasts" that may develop with oral contraceptives. Growth hormone helps promote linear growth, and low-dose testosterone therapy may be beneficial. A cardiology evaluation should be requested to assess congenital cardiac anomalies and periodically re-evaluated.

Fragile X premutation

⚒ SCIENCE REVISITED

Fragile X syndrome is caused by the expansion of a trinucleotide CGG sequence on the X chromosome. This expansion prevents the expression of the protein coded by the *FMR1* gene. Normal individuals have 29–31 CGG repeats; "intermediate" is considered 40–60 repeats. Individuals with the premutation have 55–200 repeats. This form is unstable and susceptible to expansion in offspring. Fragile X syndrome manifests with over 200 repeats and is characterized by mental retardation and macroorchidism in males. Fragile X syndrome is the most frequent inherited cause of mental retardation, with an incidence of 1 in 1,200 males and 1 in 2,000 females.

Ovarian failure or ovarian insufficiency may be presenting sign of the *FMR1* premutation in girls. Because of the implications to family members, *FMR1* screening should be obtained in all girls with primary ovarian insufficiency. If the *FMR1* premutation is identified, genetic counseling is essential to determine the risk in family members' offspring. Fragile X syndrome is the most common cause of heritable mental retardation.

Autoimmune disorders

Girls with autoimmune disorders may have a higher risk of developing ovarian insufficiency, presumably due to "oophoritis" with inflammation and destruction of oocytes. Ovarian insufficiency may be the first obvious manifestation of an autoimmune disorder, so periodic rescreening is advisable for a girl with "unexplained" primary ovarian insufficiency. If the diagnosis is uncertain, consultation with a rheumatologist is appropriate.

Swyer syndrome

⚒ SCIENCE REVISITED

Swyer syndrome—46,XY gonadal dysgenesis– is caused by a failure to form functional testes during fetal development. During normal male fetal development, testosterone secreted by the testes stimulates the internal male genital tract to form. Testosterone is converted to dihydrotestosterone (DHT) in the external genitals, and DHT is responsible for development of the external male phallus. Antimüllerian hormone (AMH) is also secreted by normal testes during fetal development, and causes regression of the müllerian ducts. In 46,XY gonadal dysgenesis, the female internal and external organs develop if the testes fail to produce testosterone and AMH. Incomplete formation of the testes can result in ambiguous genitalia.

Although Swyer syndrome is not a form of ovarian failure, it is a form of hypogonadotropic hypogonadism, and a phenotypic female presents with absent pubertal development. These girls have a high incidence of gonadal tumors, and androgen-secreting tumors will cause masculinization. Because of the potential for malignancy, gonadectomy is advised when the diagnosis of Swyer syndrome is established by the combination of elevated FSH, a phenotypic female, and a 46,XY karyotype.

"Below the waist" causes of amenorrhea

Girls with congenital anomalies of the müllerian duct system present with normal thelarche but have amenorrhea due to any of the following conditions: absence of a functional uterus with either Mayer–Rokitanksy–Kuster–Hauser syndrome or androgen insensitivity syndrome, an obstruction caused by an imperforate hymen or a transverse vaginal septum, or less commonly cervical agenesis. With obstruction, uterine bleeding occurs, but menstrual blood is trapped and distends the uterus or vagina, and each episode is increasingly painful. Retrograde menstruation promotes implantation and growth of peritoneal endometriosis. Accurate diagnosis and management are essential to relive the extreme pain due to obstruction, to help the patients with vaginal agenesis to achieve optimal sexual function, and to allow for sexual maturation but prevent gonadal tumors in patients with androgen insensitivity syndrome.

Vaginal agenesis

The differential diagnosis for a patient who presents with normal thelarche and nonobstructive amenorrhea and normal external genitalia but a small vaginal pouch includes müllerian agenesis (Mayer–Rokitanksy–Kuster–Hauser syndrome) and androgen insensitivity syndrome. Although the external genital appearance is similar, adrenarche is normal with müllerian agenesis and scant or absent with androgen insensitivity syndrome. The diagnosis is confirmed with karyotype testing, and is 46,XX with müllerian agenesis and 46,XY with androgen insensitivity syndrome.

Müllerian agenesis

Müllerian agenesis is identified by a small vaginal pouch and normal perineum on examination, and occurs in approximately 1 in 4,000–5,000 female births. It is the second most common cause of primary amenorrhea, occurring in

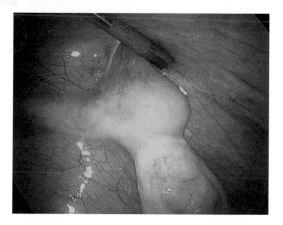

Figure 3.6 Laparoscopic image of nonfunctional rudimentary uterine horns with normal ovaries (Plate 3.6).

approximately 15% of girls with primary amenorrhea. It is caused by the absence (agenesis) of the müllerian ducts or abnormal formation (dysgenesis) of these ducts, leading to a nonfunctional rudimentary uterine horn (Figure 3.6). Renal and skeletal anomalies are commonly identified with imaging studies. Psychological counseling and support are needed, since a medical or surgical intervention is required before a girl initiates intercourse. Typical issues include an adolescent with self-image adjustments, issues with relationships and sexuality, and the inability to conceive a child naturally. However, since ovarian function is normal, pregnancy is possible with utilization of a gestational carrier.

Androgen insensitivity syndrome

> **⚗ SCIENCE REVISITED**
>
> Androgen insensitivity syndrome is caused by gene defects that cause androgen receptor abnormalities and occurs in approximately 1 in 20,000 births. Testicular development in utero is normal, and testosterone and müllerian inhibiting substance (or antimüllerian hormone) is secreted form the gonads. However, since testosterone drives the differentiation of the wolffian system into male internal genitalia, and dihydrotestosterone drives development of the external genitalia to cause male phallic differentiation,

the wolffian duct system degenerates and the external genitalia develop along female patterns in the absence of a functional androgen receptor. Antimüllerian hormone secreted by the testes in utero causes regression of the müllerian ducts, so the internal female genitalia, including the uterus, cervix, and upper vagina, fail to form. The brain feminizes in the absence of testosterone. At puberty, the testes secrete normal male testosterone levels, and testosterone is converted to estradiol by aromatization. The testosterone has no direct effect because of the faulty androgen receptors, so adrenarche and masculinization do not occur, but the estrogen formed by aromatization causes pubertal breast development.

Typical phenotypic features of androgen insensitivity syndrome include the presence of breast development, the absence or scarcity of pubic and axillary hair, and a vaginal pouch. A karyotype of 46,XY confirms the diagnosis of androgen insensitivity syndrome. Unlike Swyer syndrome, gonadal tumors rarely form during puberty, so gonadectomy is deferred until growth has been completed and breast development is complete. Following gonadectomy, hormone therapy is advisable to reduce the risk of osteoporosis related to long-term estrogen deficiency. Unlike müllerian agenesis, fertility is not possible, and the patient should be counseled to consider adoption or use of a gestational carrier and oocyte donor. Sexual identity is female, but in most cases vaginal dilatation or surgery is needed for intercourse. Psychological counseling is advisable for the patient and her family to help cope with the complex issues of personal identity, sexual identity, relationships, and fertility.

Other male pseudohermaphrodite disorders

A male pseudohermprodite refers to a genotypic male with feminization. Genitalia are "ambiguous," with male and female features in circumstances in which there is insufficient testosterone and dihydrotestosterone to cause male internal and external genital development. An example of abnormality includes early gonadal failure in utero, with partial masculinization, a form of Swyer syndrome. Girls with partial androgen insensitivity syndrome may develop varying degrees of masculinization of the external genitalia, including some sexual hair growth, partial labioscrotal fusion, and masculine skeletal development. If labioscrotal fusion has occurred and examination reveals a "flat" perineum, vaginal dilatation is not possible and surgical correction is needed before intercourse is possible. Individuals with 5-alpha reductase deficiency cannot convert testosterone to dihydrotestosterone and are feminized at birth, but high testosterone levels during puberty cause masculinization. As these individuals can develop into fertile males after puberty, prepubertal sexual assignment should be male.

Treatment of vaginal agenesis

The goal of treatment of individuals with vaginal agenesis is to prepare for intercourse. Whatever approach is chosen, the final outcome will be most successful in a highly motivated patient, since vaginal dilatation is needed for the most commonly utilized methods. Because of the need for the patient's participation in the process, implementation should be delayed until she is ready to begin. However, due to the sensitive emotional nature of the dilatation or surgery as a prelude to sexual debut, the legal age of 18 before which parental consent is required, and reliance on parental insurance, teenagers are placed in an awkward situation of requiring parental knowledge and approval before treatment is initiated. Psychological counseling before, during, and after treatment should be considered an integral component of the management.

Vaginal dilatation

Vaginal dilatation with the Ingram method is the procedure of choice when a vaginal pouch is present. A motivated woman will be able to have intercourse after a few weeks.

> ★ TIPS & TRICKS
>
> Initially, a short narrow dilator is positioned against the perineum, and the patient is instructed to apply her weight gradually onto a bicycle seat stool and is left in place for

approximately 30 minutes. After dilatation has been completed with the first dilator, the process is continued with longer and wider dilators until a satisfactory width and depth have been achieved.

Vecchietti vaginoplasty

The Vecchietti vaginoplasty is a surgical approach that has gained popularity in the last decade. It is a method of vaginal dilatation that is accomplished by applying progressive tension on abdominal sutures that are attached to an olive-shaped device at the perineum (Figure 3.7). It is appropriate when passive dilatation is unsuccessful, the patient is physically and emotionally prepared for surgery, and intercourse anticipated in the not too distant future. It may also be the primary approach considered if laparoscopy or laparotomy is indicated for other indications. Intercourse is possible 20 days after the olive has been removed. Long-term sexual satisfaction is greater than 80%, and results are comparable to those of vaginal dilatation and McIndoe vaginoplasty.

★ TIPS & TRICKS

Special instruments are needed to perform the Vecchietti vaginoplasty: a 2.2 × 1.9 cm acrylic "olive," an abdominal traction device, a long perineum suture-passer, and an alligator-jaw needle-passer. A laparoscopy is performed and a second port placed above the symphysis. The olive is placed at the vaginal pouch, and the sutures are placed through the vagina, into the abdomen, and through to the abdominal skin. The free ends of the sutures are attached to a traction device, and the tension is adjusted every 1–2 days. Traction placed on the sutures dilates the vagina by pulling the olive deeper into the vaginal pouch. A depth of 7–10 cm is achieved in 7–9 days. After the sutures have been removed, a soft latex 10 × 1.5 cm dilator is used continuously for 8–10 hours for 1 month. The patient then gradually advances to larger dilators of 2.0 cm and 2.5 cm diameter.

McIndoe vaginoplasty

With the McIndoe vaginoplasty, surgery is performed to create the vagina. Historically, this has been the primary surgical approach when dilatation has been unsuccessful or not possible, as may be the case for a patient with a flat perineum. Intercourse is possible within 8 weeks of surgery. Approximately 75% of women are able to achieve orgasm, and long-term satisfaction is greater than 80%.

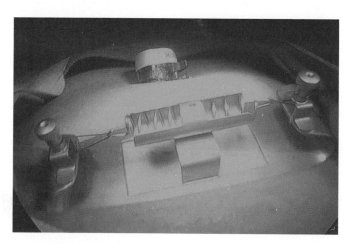

Figure 3.7 Vecchietti vaginoplasty traction device placed on the abdomen. Traction on the sutures pulls the "olive" deeper into the vaginal pouch.

The McIndoe vaginoplasty is started by making a transverse incision at the apex of the vaginal pouch. The neovaginal space is bluntly dissected, and the median raphe, a connective tissue band between bladder and rectum, is divided. The dissection is continued until the surgeon can comfortably place two fingers into the vagina. Once meticulous hemostasis is achieved, a sterile $10 \times 10 \times 20$ cm foam rubber form is cut to shape, compressed in a sterile condom, and allowed to expand in the neovaginal space. A 15–18 cm split-thickness skin graft is taken from the buttock, and the graft is sewn over the form with the skin surface touching the form. A suprapubic catheter is placed to keep pressure off of the form. The form and graft are placed into the vagina, and the edges sutured to the skin. Strict bed rest is required for 1 week to allow the graft to attach. After 1 week, the form is removed and the graft inspected. After discharge from the hospital, the foam rubber form is worn continuously for 2–4 weeks and then nightly. After the vagina has completed healing, rigid dilatation is necessary until the patient is ready to initiate sex.

It is important to emphasize that there is no "one size fits all" approach for the patient with vaginal agenesis. The patient must be ready and motivated to achieve optimal results. Those who choose surgery must realize that surgery does not avoid the need for vaginal dilatation. Most importantly, if surgery is performed, it is essential to "get it right" the first time, as scarring from suboptimal surgical outcomes can be very difficult to correct.

Obstruction and amenorrhea

Vaginal obstruction and amenorrhea is caused by one of three conditions: imperforate hymen, a transverse vaginal septum, or cervical agenesis. All of these conditions present similarly, with progressive pain at the time of expected menarche caused by uterine bleeding and distension of the obstructed organ with blood. Pain typically increases with each menses, and is most severe when the potential for gradual distention is least. Therefore, since the uterus is less distensible than the vagina, a girl with cervical agenesis will tend to have earlier and more severe cramping and pain than a girl with an imperforate hymen or a low transverse vaginal septum. The correct diagnosis is based on the clinical history, physical examination, ultrasound, and MRI studies when the diagnosis has not been established with certainty.

The examination of a girl with "outlet" obstruction may be obvious. For example, an imperforate hymen is thin, translucent, and bulging. A transverse vaginal septum is nontranslucent; a mass caused by distention of the upper vagina with blood (a hematocolpos) may be palpable if the patient is cooperative, but it may be challenging to gain the cooperation of a young adolescent girl who is experiencing excruciating pain. For this reason, abdominal ultrasound examination should be able to differentiate the patient with a high transverse vaginal septum from the patient with cervical agenesis: with a septum, a hematocolpos is identified, with or without distention of the cervix and uterus with blood, whereas only the distended uterus will be seen with cervical agenesis.

The management of an imperforate hymen is performed in the operating suite with sedation, although it can be performed in the emergency center if the patient is cooperative and can be sedated. A cruciate incision is made in the hymen to allow the escape of blood and the edges can be trimmed if excessive tissue is present, and sutured if bleeding.

The management of a transverse vaginal septum is more challenging and ideally should be performed by a physician with experience and training with similar procedures. Preoperative MRI helps to determine the extent of the septum. A high transverse vaginal septum can be difficult to enter though a lower vaginal incision, and dissection can be carried too far anteriorly or posteriorly. Intraoperative abdominal ultrasound can help keep the surgeon in the proper plane. If there is a large gap between the upper and lower vaginal segments, it may be necessary to perform a split-thickness skin graft. Vaginal dilatation is required after surgical correction of a transverse vaginal septum to prevent stenosis, which can cause obstruction or dyspareunia.

An MRI scan is essential to properly evaluate the adolescent with suspected cervical agenesis, since repair is considered feasible if the cervix is present. Most authorities recommend hysterectomy if the cervix is absent, as there have been deaths reported from ascending infections following surgical creation of a cervix. However, there have been a few cases reported with successful repairs in referral centers. If the diagnosis is in doubt and the physician or family wish to delay difficult decision-making, it is reasonable to prescribe continuous hormonal contraception to suppress menses and limit recurrent pain. With this approach, definitive therapy may be postponed indefinitely in most patients.

★ TIPS & TRICKS

Since vaginal dilatation is recommended after correction of a high transverse vaginal septum and most girls present near the time of expected menarche, many patients lack the motivation or maturity to comply with a regimen requiring years of vaginal dilatation before initiating intercourse. We have used a regimen of drainage and rinsing of the hematocolpos with a large-bore bone marrow aspiration needle under heavy sedation using abdominal ultrasound and broad-spectrum antibiotics, and then suppressing menstruation with continuous hormonal contraception or long-term use of a gonadotropin-releasing hormone agonist with low-dose hormone therapy. When the patient is motivated to begin vaginal dilatation, vaginal dilatation helps to distend the lower vagina to shorten the gap between the vaginal segments and greatly simplifies the surgical repair.

Evaluation of delayed puberty

The evaluation of delayed puberty is initiated considering the differential diagnoses. For simplicity, if the patient's examination reveals a normal cervix and vagina, the physician can divide the differential diagnosis into "above the neck" and "below the neck" causes. The diagnosis of a congenital anomaly is obvious if a vaginal pouch, flat perineum, or hematocolpos is identified.

Historical features help identify specific causes. The physician should elicit a history of head trauma or trauma at birth, assess growth charts to determine if slow growth is progressing, determine a family history of pubertal delay, ovarian failure, and mental retardation, and determine whether the patient has a history of chronic illness, eating disorder, or extreme athleticism. A history of pubertal milestones should be determined for onset, progress, and the age and stage of arrested development.

A comprehensive examination is performed, including examination of the genitalia. Important components of the assessment should include determination of olfaction (absent with Kallman syndrome), height and weight measurements, upper and lower segment lengths (which vary with Turner syndrome and other anomalies), and arm span. Tanner staging should be assessed, but this should include measurement of the diameter of breast tissue, examination for galactorrhea, and description of pubic hair growth. Since CNS and pituitary tumors are in the initial differential diagnosis, optic discs and visual fields should be assessed. The finding of hemitemporal hemianopsia visual field defects suggests compression of the bifurcation of the optic nerve from a pituitary mass.

★ TIPS & TRICKS

Laboratory assessment of delayed puberty or pubertal arrest begins with a follicle-stimulating hormone (FSH) level. An elevated level indicates a "below the neck" cause: ovarian failure or primary ovarian insufficiency, both terms reflecting follicle and oocyte depletion. A karyotype should be obtained if the FSH is elevated to assess for Turner syndrome and the presence of a Y chromosome. A pelvic ultrasound should be performed to assess for the presence of follicles and determine whether an adnexal mass is present. An autoimmune evaluation is initiated if the karyotype fails to provide an explanation for the accelerated depletion of follicles.

A normal or low FSH level indicates an "above the neck" etiology as long as the pelvic examination is normal. A pelvic ultrasound provides a wealth of information regarding the presence or absence of ovarian follicles, an assessment of the endometrial thickness, and an initial screening for anomalies. Other laboratory tests should include thyroid-stimulating hormone and free thyroxine to assess thyroid dysfunction, and prolactin to screen for a pituitary adenoma. Unless a clear etiology is identified, a pituitary MRI should be performed to assess for the presence of a pituitary or CNS lesion. A GnRH stimulation test is sometimes useful to assess the maturation of the HPO axis, and a bone age can determine if further growth is expected.

Conclusions

Puberty is a dynamic and complex phase associated with many different abnormalities that manifest as disorders of menstruation. In order to deal with these unusual but potentially dangerous conditions, the physician must maintain a uniform approach to the underlying differential diagnoses. An approach that emphasizes simplicity, with "above the neck" and "below the neck" causes of precocious and delayed puberty, can help the provider organize the evaluation, especially when initiating an assessment of unusual condition. If the diagnosis and solutions are not obvious, the provider may serve the patient and family best by referral to a provider with extensive experience with pubertal disorders.

Selected bibliography

Houk CP, Kunselman AR, Lee PA. The diagnostic value of a brief GnRH analogue stimulation test in girls with central precocious puberty: a single 30-minute post-stimulation LH sample is adequate. J Ped Endocrinol 2008;21:1113–18.

Hurst BS, Rock JA. Preoperative dilatation to facilitate repair of the high transverse vaginal septum. Fertil Steril 1992;57:1351–3.

Kadir RA, Lukes AS, Kouides PA, Fernandez H, Goudemand J. Management of excessive menstrual bleeding in women with hemostatic disorders. Fertil Steril 2005;84:1352–9.

Karnis MF, Zimon AE, Lalwani SI, Timmreck LS, Klipstein S, Reindollar RH. Risk of death in pregnancy achieved through oocyte donation in patients with Turner syndrome: a national survey. Fertil Steril 2003;80:498–501.

Kouides PA, Conard J, Peyvandi F, Lukes A, Kadir R. Hemostasis and menstruation: appropriate investigation for underlying disorders of hemostasis in women with excessive menstrual bleeding. Fertil Steril 2005;84: 1345–51.

Laughlin GA, Dominguez CE, Yen SS. Nutritional and endocrine-metabolic aberrations in women with functional hypothalamic amenorrhea. J Clin Endocrinol Metab 1998;83:25–32.

Lee PA, Houk CP. Gonadotropin-releasing hormone analog therapy for central precocious puberty and other childhood disorders affecting growth and puberty. Treat Endocrinol 2006;5:287–96.

Migeon CJ, Wisneiewski AB. Congenital adrenal hyperplasia owing to 21-hydroxylase deficiency: growth, development, and therapeutic considerations. Endocrinol Metab Clin N Am 2001;30:193–206.

Nelson LM. Clinical practice. Primary ovarian insufficiency. N Engl J Med 2009;360:606–14.

Oakes MB, Eyvazzadeh AD, Quint E, Smith YR. Complete androgen insensitivity syndrome–a review. J Ped Adolesc Gynecol 2008;21: 305–10.

Practice Committee of the American Society for Reproductive Medicine. Current evaluation of amenorrhea. Fertil Steril 2006;86:S148–55.

Sybert VP, McCauley E. Turner's syndrome. N Engl J Med 2004;351:1227–38.

Trakakis E, Loghis C, Kassanos D. Congenital adrenal hyperplasia because of 21-hydroxylase deficiency. A genetic disorder of interest to obstetricians and gynecologists. Obstet Gynecol Surv 2009;64:177–89.

Troiano RN, McCarthy SM. Mullerian duct anomalies: imaging and clinical issues. Radiology 2004;233:19–34.

4

Menstrual Disorders During the Reproductive Years

Michelle L. Matthews

Carolinas Medical Center, Charlotte, North Carolina, USA

Introduction

Abnormalities in menstrual function are a common condition seen by gynecologists and primary healthcare providers. Approximately 1 in 20 women present for evaluation and treatment of heavy menstrual bleeding each year, and 20% of all women obtain a hysterectomy for heavy bleeding by age 60 years. Over one third of hysterectomies are performed for bleeding unrelated to any uterine pathology, indicating that other etiologies are common. Irregular vaginal bleeding is certainly a health concern for women that can significantly impact quality of life.

The menstrual cycle will be between 24 and 35 days in length. The first day of the cycle is considered the first day of full bleeding. The usual duration is 4–5 days of bleeding, but the range is 2–7 days. The usual volume of bleed loss is approximately 30 mL, and greater than 80 mL is considered abnormal. Abnormal menstrual bleeding may present as heavy bleeding occurring at regular menstrual intervals (menorrhagia), as bleeding that occurs at irregular intervals with normal or reduced flow (metrorrhagia), or as both irregular intervals and excessive volume and duration of flow (menometrorrhagia). Other menstrual abnormalities include polymenorrhea (cycles every 24 days or more frequently), oligomenorrhea (cycle length over 35 days), and amenorrhea (absence of menstruation of at least three cycles).

Abnormalities in menstrual function can occur from a variety of etiologies regardless of the presentation. Generally, most irregular vaginal bleeding is secondary to either a hormonal etiology or a structural abnormality of the uterus. Bleeding may also arise from many other causes, including systemic diseases and coagulopathies. It is important for healthcare providers to have an organized approach to evaluation and treatment given the variety of presentations and etiologies for abnormal bleeding.

Causes of abnormal bleeding

The differential diagnosis for abnormal uterine bleeding is extensive but may be organized into two primary categories: bleeding due to structural abnormalities of the reproductive tract (benign conditions and malignancies), and other nonstructural etiologies (Table 4.1). Nonstructural causes of menstrual disturbances are often related to anovulatory bleeding secondary to both pathologic and physiologic causes. Although less common, other etiologies should also be considered, such as systemic disease, iatrogenic causes, and pregnancy-related bleeding.

Structural abnormalities of the uterus

Benign uterine conditions

Fibroids, adenomyosis, and polyps are benign lesions of the uterus and a common cause of abnormal uterine bleeding. Fibroids are the most

Disorders of Menstruation, 1st edition. Edited by Paul B. Marshburn and Bradley S. Hurst.
© 2011 Blackwell Publishing Ltd.

Table 4.1 Causes of menstrual disorders

Structural conditions of the uterus
Benign
• Fibroids • Endometriosis • Adenomyosis • Polyps
Malignancies
• Endometrial hyperplasia • Endometrial cancer • Estrogen-secreting neoplasms • Cervical cancer • Vaginal or vulvar cancer
Other anatomic causes
• Endometritis • Cervicitis • Trauma • Foreign body • Condyloma • Ulceration • Genitourinary (hematuria, urethral diverticulum) • Gastrointestinal (hemorrhoids, inflammatory bowel diseases)
Hormonal (anovulation)
Physiologic
• Puberty • Perimenopause
Pathologic
• Hypothalamic • Pituitary (hyperprolactinemia) • Thyroid • Polycystic ovarian syndrome
Other causes
Liver disease
Renal disease
Coagulopathies
Iatrogenic (medications, chemotherapy)
Pregnancy-related bleeding
Trauma

common pelvic tumor in women. They are found in approximately one third of reproductive-age women and over 50% of hysterectomy specimens. Abnormal bleeding occurs in approximately 30% of patients with fibroids. The size and location of the fibroids often impact their clinical presentation. Fibroids that are located in the cavity of the uterus (intracavitary) or impinge on the cavity of the uterus (submucosal) are most likely to present with irregular bleeding. Larger fibroids in the myometrial wall (intramural) are also associated with irregular bleeding.

Menorrhagia is a common symptom; however, irregular bleeding and intermenstrual spotting are often earlier presenting symptoms.

Adenomyosis is a condition in which endometrial glands and stroma invade the myometrium. Although the etiology is unclear, the condition may result in dysmenorrhea, dyspareunia, and irregular bleeding. The symptoms often present similarly to endometriosis. Bleeding tends to be cyclic, prolonged, and heavy, similar to the bleeding pattern with fibroids.

Endometrial polyps are another common benign lesion of the uterus. They result from excessive growth of endometrial tissue inside the cavity of the uterus. Their presentation may vary depending on the size of the polyp. Small polyps may present with intermenstrual or postcoital bleeding, while larger polyps may present with menorrhagia.

Gynecologic malignancies

Malignancies of the cervix, uterus, fallopian tubes, vagina, and vulva are relatively uncommon in reproductive-age women but any may present with irregular bleeding. The two most common cancers to present in women of reproductive age are endometrial cancer and cervical cancer. Fortunately, the incidence of cervical cancer is decreasing with the use of cervical screening. In addition, the implementation of vaccinations for women for common human papillomavirus subtypes that increase the risk of cancer (subtypes 16 and 18) will continue to decrease the incidence of the disease. Irregular bleeding, particularly postcoital bleeding, is a common presenting symptom of cervical cancer and warrants further investigation with visual examination, pap smear and colposcopy when indicated based on the Papanicolau smear results.

The risk of endometrial cancer increases with age. The risk for women age 30–34 years is 2 per 100,000 women, for age 35–39 it is 6 per 100,000 women, and in the perimenopause it is 4 per 10,000 women. Endometrial hyperplasia is the precursor to endometrial cancer. The risk is increased for premenopausal women with unopposed estrogen exposure either through exogenous use or estrogen-secreting tumors, and for women with anovulatory cycles and excess estrogen exposure (e.g., polycystic ovarian syndrome [PCOS]).

Other anatomic causes of nonuterine bleeding

There are a variety of anatomic causes of nonuterine bleeding that must be considered in the evaluation of abnormal bleeding. The cervix, vagina, and vulva may bleed in response to trauma, foreign bodies, atrophy, infection, condylomas, ulceration, and endometriosis. It is also important to remember nongynecologic causes of bleeding such as bleeding from the urinary tract (hematuria, urethral diverticulum) and gastrointestinal bleeding (hemorrhoids, fissures, inflammatory bowel disease). Patient history of other medical conditions and close examination will help identify these conditions.

Hormonal etiologies of abnormal menstrual bleeding

The vast majority of hormonally related abnormal uterine bleeding is secondary to anovulation and a subsequent imbalance of estrogen and progesterone. This typically results in bleeding secondary to estrogen withdrawal, or estrogen breakthrough or progesterone breakthrough bleeding. These causes are outlined in Table 4.2.

In order to understand the mechanism of abnormal bleeding, it is important to review the process of normal menstruation. Menstruation is the cyclic shedding of the endometrial lining of the uterus in response to withdrawal of estrogen and progesterone in the absence of pregnancy. Withdrawal of progesterone results in changes in the endometrial vessels, tissue necrosis, and bleeding. A variety of local mediators are involved in the complex process of endometrial stability. Perhaps the most important of these are prostaglandins, which are released in response to progesterone withdrawal. Prostaglandins appear to be involved in the vascular and myometrial changes that occur at menstruation. Most of the tissue is shed in 1–2 days, but bleeding continues for several days until new tissue is generated from the basal layer of the endometrium in response to estrogen. Whereas normal menstruation occurs by withdrawal of estrogen and progesterone, bleeding can occur in response to a fall in estrogen alone or progesterone alone.

Table 4.2 Anovulatory uterine bleeding

Bleeding due to estrogen withdrawal (lack of estrogen)
Discontinuation of hormonal therapy
Bilateral oophorectomy
Midcycle drop in estradiol after ovulation
Excessive exercise
Eating disorders
Bleeding due to estrogen breakthrough (chronic unopposed estrogen with no progesterone)
Polycystic ovarian syndrome
Unopposed estrogen hormonal therapy
Bleeding due to progesterone-breakthrough (high progesterone to estrogen ratio)
Progesterone-only contraceptives
Combined estrogen–progesterone oral contraceptives

⚙ SCIENCE REVISITED

Hormonal bleeding is a result of estrogen and/or progesterone withdrawal from the endometrium. This results in shedding of the functional layer of the uterus, leaving the basalis layer to regenerate endometrium. Shedding of the endometrium occurs through a complex sequence of events that includes enzymatic degeneration of the functional layer of the uterus. Enzymatic autodigestion results from several mechanisms triggered by estrogen and progesterone withdrawal, including release of lysosomal enzymes, proteases, and inflammatory cells.

Plasmin is released to prevent clotting of menstrual fluid to form a base on the denuded endometrial tissue. Menstrual bleeding stops as the spiral arterioles in the basal layer of the endometrium vasoconstrict in response to high concentrations of prostaglandins in the menstrual fluid. As estradiol rises during the early follicular phase, thrombosis of denuded vessels occurs that also helps stop menstrual flow. The uterine stroma regenerates from cells located in the basal layer of the endometrium, and numerous growth factors appear to aid in this process. As the uterine endometrium regenerates, the menstrual cycle ceases until the late luteal phase, when the cycle starts again in response falling levels of estrogen and progesterone as the corpus luteum regresses.

Although the underlying mechanisms controlling menstruation are complex, it is important to remember that most irregular bleeding is prevented by the balance of estrogen and progesterone induced by ovulation. In a normal menstrual cycle, gonadotropin-releasing hormone (GnRH) from the hypothalamus signals the release of follicle-stimulating hormone (FSH) from the pituitary, which then results in ovarian stimulation of estradiol production. Ovulation is triggered through complex signaling pathways resulting in progesterone production by the ovary. Anovulatory cycles are the result of abnormalities in the normal hormonal signals between the hypothalamus, pituitary, and ovary. Anovulatory bleeding may be due to either a normal physiologic process or a pathologic condition.

Physiologic anovulation

Irregular bleeding is a normal physiologic process at the beginning of reproductive function at puberty, and toward the end of menstrual function at menopause. Abnormal menstrual bleeding is common secondary to anovulatory cycles, which may occur intermittently for 2–5 years during these transitions. The age of the patient is an important factor when considering whether the irregular bleeding is a normal process. Certainly, the first few years of menstruation are common considerations. The average age of first menstruation is 10–12 years, but the normal range may be 8–16 years.

Perimenopause is the interval before menopause and is marked by the onset of menstrual irregularity. The age range of the perimenopausal transition is 39–51 years, with a median age of 47.5 years and a duration of approximately 4–5 years. Elevated FSH levels early in the menstrual cycle accelerate ovarian follicle maturation. The average follicular phase decreases by 3–4 days, so menstrual cycle lengths shorten because the follicular phase of the cycle is the major determinant of cycle length. Conversely, some cycles may be anovulatory, resulting in missed menses or a longer cycle length. The effect of shorter cycles combined with sporadic longer cycles results in a pattern of unpredictable, irregular bleeding. As menopause approaches, more cycles become anovulatory and cycle lengths increase.

Pathologic anovulation

In addition to normal physiologic processes that result in anovulation and irregular bleeding, there are several pathologic processes with a similar presentation. Pathologic causes such as hypothalamic or pituitary dysfunction, hypothyroidism, PCOS, premature ovarian failure, and systemic and iatrogenic causes must be considered.

Hypothalamic disorders may result in abnormal GnRH release and a subsequent decrease in pituitary secretion of gonadotropins. The net result is failure of ovarian stimulation and estrogen production. This typically results in abnormal bleeding that is light and irregular. Common causes of hypothalamic dysfunction include excessive exercise, eating disorders, and stress. However, a neoplasm should be suspected if there is no other obvious etiology of a hypothalamic disorder, and imaging is warranted with magnetic resonance imaging.

Pituitary disorders result in irregular bleeding secondary to anovulation. The most common pituitary disorder is hyperprolactinemia, which is a result of the oversecretion of prolactin from the pituitary. Hyperprolatinemia results in suppression of GnRH from the hypothalamus by stimulating dopamine release from the arcuate nucleus of the hypothalamus. The most common cause of hyperprolactinemia is a prolactinoma. Most prolactinomas are microadenomas measuring less than 10 mm. Larger macroadenomas may also present with headaches and bitemporal hemianopsia secondary to optic nerve compression. Most prolactinomas present without any symptoms other than galactorrhea and/or menstrual irregularity. There are many other causes of hyperprolactinemia including medication (narcotics, dopamine antagonists, neuroleptics, antidepressants), systemic disease (renal failure, liver disease), neurogenic (chest wall lesions), endocrine disease (primary hypothyroidism, Cushing disease, PCOS), and suprasellar disorders including tumors. Menstrual function will often return to normal by medically correcting the hyperprolactinemia with dopamine agonists (bromocriptine, cabergoline).

Thyroid disease may result in menstrual disturbances and subsequent irregular bleeding. Hyperthyroidism generally results in light irregular bleeding and eventual amenorrhea. In the early stages, however, it can present with mild irregular bleeding. Hypothyroidism is more likely to result in menorrhagia and weight gain. Treatment of the underlying thyroid disease will often correct the menstrual irregularity.

PCOS commonly presents with irregular menstruation secondary to anovulation. Patients with PCOS have several etiologies for anovulation including disordered luteinizing hormone (LH) and FSH release as well as elevated androgens that suppress ovulation. Although there is no universally accepted definition of the diagnostic criteria required to make the diagnosis of PCOS, the most commonly accepted criteria include a combination of two of three of the following: clinical or biochemical evidence of elevated androgens, polycystic ovaries on ultrasound, and oligo- or anovulation. Other endocrinopathies such as diabetes mellitus, Cushing syndrome, and congenital adrenal hyperplasia may also present with abnormal uterine bleeding and a similar presentation to PCOS.

Although it is a less common cause, patients with premature ovarian failure present with amenorrhea prior to the age of 35 years. The onset may be abrupt, but more often it is more gradual in onset, presenting first with irregular bleeding. Typically, the bleeding is light and irregular. The ovarian failure is represented by low estradiol production, elevated FSH, and anovulation. The etiologies are often idiopathic but may be constitutional or the result of gonadal dysgenesis or an autoimmune condition. Patients may also complain other sequelae of hypoestrogenism such as vaginal atrophy, hot flashes, mood swings, and insomnia.

Other etiologies of irregular bleeding

Systemic disease

Abnormal bleeding may be one of the presenting symptoms in a patient with a serious systemic disease. The most common systemic diseases resulting in irregular menstrual function are liver disease, renal disease, and inherited or acquired coagulopathies. Hepatic dysfunction results in abnormal production of fibrinogen and clotting factors, in addition to its impact on estrogen bioavailability by the production of sex hormone-binding globulin. The combination of the impact on clotting factors and estrogen availability may result in irregular bleeding. The kidneys are responsible for the excretion of estrogen and progesterone. Renal disease impacts the amount of circulating hormones and thereby impacts ovulation and menstruation.

Although most bleeding disorders will present in adolescents with menorrhagia, it is important to consider undiagnosed coagulopathies in all reproductive-aged women presenting with menorrhagia with no obvious anatomic etiology. A significant family history of a bleeding diathesis warrants further evaluation. A history of epistaxis and easy bruising may be helpful, but these do not appear to be clear discriminatory markers of an inherited coagulopathy. Therefore, testing should be performed if a suspicion exists in a patient with menorrhagia. The most common acquired bleeding disorders include leukemias and acquired platelet disorders. The most common platelet disorder is idiopathic thrombocytopenic purpura and can be detected with a platelet count. The incidence of platelet abnormalities is as high as 50% in patients with severe unexplained menorrhagia.

Although it may also be acquired, the most common inherited bleeding disorder is von Willebrand disease. Patients with Von Willebrand disease have decreased coagulation factor VII levels and the von Willebrand factor. Although the prevalence of von Willebrand disease in the general population is reported to be approximately 1%, the prevalence in women presenting with menorrhagia ranges and may be as high as 20%. Other factor deficiencies occur very infrequently.

Unfortunately, there is no consensus opinion of what specific testing should be ordered to evaluate for coagulopathies, and testing recommendations vary based on ethnic background and history. Testing is expensive and is not warranted for all women with irregular bleeding, given the relatively high incidence of the condition. Preliminary testing often includes assessment of platelet count, ristocetin cofactor assay for von Willebrand factor function, and a partial thromboplastin time and prothrombin time. However, testing can be difficult and should be performed by laboratories specializing in coagulation disorders. If a coagulopathy is suspected, it may be most prudent to refer the patient to a hematologist for the most appropriate evaluation. Patient history is important in determining whether further evaluation is warranted. Further evaluation should be considered if the patient history is significant for one of four key elements: a duration of menses greater than or equal to 7 days and either "flooding" or impairment of daily activities with most periods, a history of treatment of anemia, a family history of a diagnosed bleeding disorder, or excessive bleeding with tooth extraction, childbirth, miscarriage, or surgery.

Iatrogenic

It is important to consider iatrogenic causes of abnormal uterine bleeding if no other etiology is determined. Certain medications have been associated with irregular uterine bleeding, particularly hormonal medications (estrogens, progestins, oral contraceptives, hormone replacement therapy, tamoxifen). In fact, breakthrough bleeding is a common side effect of these medications, particularly in the first few months of use. Other medications have been associated with irregular bleeding, such as centrally acting agents (psychotropic agents, antidepressants), antihypertensives, dopamine antagonists, and anticoagulants. Prior radiation and chemotherapy may also impact ovarian and pituitary function, resulting in irregular bleeding.

Pregnancy-related bleeding

Pregnancy-related vaginal bleeding occurs relatively frequently, particularly in early pregnancy: approximately 20–40% of patients will have first-trimester bleeding. The chance of clinically recognized pregnancy loss increases with age and may be as high as 20%. Bleeding often resolves spontaneously with expectant management, and an etiology may not always be determined. Common known causes of bleeding include fetal demise, subchorionic hemorrhage, and abortion (incomplete, complete, threatened, inevitable). Other less common causes include ectopic pregnancy and gestational trophoblastic disease.

Ultrasound assessment and quantitative human chorionic gonadotropin (hCG) measurement are the most helpful tests in determining the etiology of the bleeding and the most appropriate treatment plan. Ultrasound may identify a subchorionic hemorrhage visualized between the gestational sac and the uterine wall. A subchorionic hemorrhage may resolve spontaneously with expectant management, and its resolution may be followed using serial ultrasounds. A diagnosis of a nonviable pregnancy may be made by ultrasound if fetal cardiac activity is not present when it had been visualized previously, or if cardiac activity is absent in an embryo with a crown–rump length greater than 5 mm. Other signs of a nonviable pregnancy include absence of a fetal pole when the mean gestational sac diameter is greater than 18 mm on transvaginal ultrasound.

Measurement of serum hCG is also helpful in evaluation of early pregnancy viability, particularly if ultrasound is inconclusive. Serial measurements of hCG should be evaluated at 48-hour intervals. Declining hCG concentrations, or hCG that does not increase by 66% over 2 days may be indicative of a nonviable pregnancy (intrauterine or ectopic). It is important to remember, however, that patients with multiple pregnancies may have one ongoing viable pregnancy even though another gestation is nonviable. Therefore, caution should be used when interpreting serial hCG results when there is a suspicion of multiple pregnancy (e.g., a patient on ovulation induction therapy).

Ultrasound and hCG are also helpful in diagnosing gestational trophoblastic disease. Gestational trophoblastic diseases include a variety of related conditions arising from the placenta, including molar pregnancies, gestational choriocarcinomas, and placental site trophoblastic tumors. These entities are histologically distinct but often present similarly with abnormal uterine bleeding and a positive pregnancy test. Patients often present with abnormally high hCG concentrations and ultrasound findings of a diffuse echogenic pattern. A viable fetus may very rarely be identified. The final diagnosis is confirmed based on pathologic specimen analysis, and treatment depends on histology. Depending on the specific gestational trophoblastic disease, therapy may include surgery and/or chemotherapy. Therefore, patients should be referred accordingly for evaluation and treatment.

Evaluation of irregular bleeding

Patients with bothersome unpredictable bleeding, frequent cycles, and/or heavy bleeding are often a diagnostic and therapeutic challenge. Anovulatory bleeding should be considered a diagnosis of exclusion as it is essential to rule out all other causes of abnormal bleeding before initiating therapy for presumed anovulation. A history of ovulatory symptoms such as dysmenorrhea, premenstrual symptoms, breast tenderness, and bloating may help differentiate ovulatory from anovulatory bleeding.

A thorough menstrual history should be elicited, and menstrual blood loss should be quantified. It is important to remember that a woman's perception of her menstrual flow is often unreliable as menstrual blood loss is difficult to quantify. However, patients are often more able to detect a change in their cycle length, volume of flow, or duration. A thorough history should include inquiry into medical conditions that may contribute to abnormal bleeding (coagulation disorders, liver disease, thyroid disease, prolactin disorders). Patients should be questioned for other causes of bleeding including medications (anticoagulants, hormonal), infections, foreign bodies (intrauterine contraceptive device [IUD]), trauma, and any history of reproductive tract conditions (leiomyomas, endometrial polyps, endometrial hyperplasia, carcinoma). Pregnancy and complications of pregnancy including miscarriage must also be considered. Endometrial hyperplasia and subsequent endometrial carcinoma are concerns in the perimenopause secondary to the periods of hyperestrogenism. A history of obesity, nulliparity, and diabetes increases the risk of endometrial cancer.

A general physical and pelvic examination should be performed. The physical examination should include abdominal palpation for evidence of masses, ascites, or an enlarged liver or spleen, indicating evidence of malignancy. Enlarged lymph nodes may suggest tumor or infection. Bruising or bleeding may indicate a coagulopathy. Cardiovascular and breast examinations should also be performed. The pelvic examination should include examination of the external genitalia as well as urethra, vagina, and cervix for evidence of lesions, atrophy, polyps, ulcers, or masses. A complete bimanual examination includes evaluation of the uterus for size, contour, and tenderness, as well as evaluation of the adnexa for masses. An enlarged uterus may indicate leiomyomas, adenomyosis, or pregnancy. A rectal examination for occult blood and a cervical Papanicolau smear should be obtained.

The history and physical examination with help identify the likely underlying etiology of the bleeding. Evaluation should be tailored to the patient's presentation but generally includes laboratory testing, imaging studies, and occasionally more invasive testing with endometrial biopsy or surgery. Infrequent and light cycles or midcycle spotting are rarely the result of a neoplastic process of the uterus. Menses that are significantly increased in flow or duration should be evaluated by endometrial biopsy and/or uterine imaging studies. Patients with a long-standing history of anovulation are at particular risk of endometrial hyperplasia and endometrial carcinoma. Dilatation and curettage (D&C) has been considered the "gold standard." However, less invasive methods have been advocated to evaluate uterine pathology. These include transvaginal sonography (TVS), saline infusion sonography (SIS), and/or endometrial biopsy. These should be performed prior to medical management if risk factors exist, or after a trial of medical management if bleeding persists.

Laboratory testing

A complete blood count, pregnancy test, and blood chemistry should be ordered, as well as thyroid and prolactin levels (Figure 4.1). Coagulation tests are indicated in patients with a history of bleeding tendencies or easy bruisability. Additional hormonal testing of FSH and estradiol is particularly helpful in the evaluation of a hormonal etiology of abnormal menstrual bleeding. FSH and estradiol should be drawn in the early follicular phase of the cycle (day 2–3) to be interpreted properly. Basal FSH values drawn during menstrual day 2–3 have been the routinely utilized as a marker of ovarian function.

As FSH values increase, ovarian responsiveness decreases and cycles become irregular. The cutoff value used to define a "normal" FSH may vary between laboratories. An FSH value of 10–15 IU/L is generally considered borderline, and values over 15 IU/L are considered elevated and may correlate with menstrual irregularities. It is important when assessing FSH values to also evaluate basal estradiol as an elevation may suppress FSH and give a falsely reassuring value. A normal basal estradiol may vary between laboratories but typically is less than 60 pg/mL.

Both low FSH and low estradiol levels may indicate a hypothalamic component of menstrual irregularity that may not otherwise be obvious from patient history (e.g., excessive exercise, eating disorders). In these cases, another etiology should be considered, such as Kallmann syndrome or an intracranial lesion. Kallmann syndrome patients may also present with anosmia as the underlying defect is related to failure of migration of GnRH-releasing cells from the olfactory placode during fetal development. Genetic testing is available to confirm the diagnosis, although many patients with presumed Kallmann syndrome do not have a detectable genetic mutation in the Kallmann gene (*KAL1*).

Patients with PCOS often present with low to normal FSH and slightly elevated estradiol secondary to increased peripheral circulation of estrogens. Laboratory testing of FSH and estradiol helps identify patients with a nonclassic presentation for PCOS such as lean variants or patients without manifestations of androgen excess. Another etiology of a high estradiol and

Abnormal Bleeding

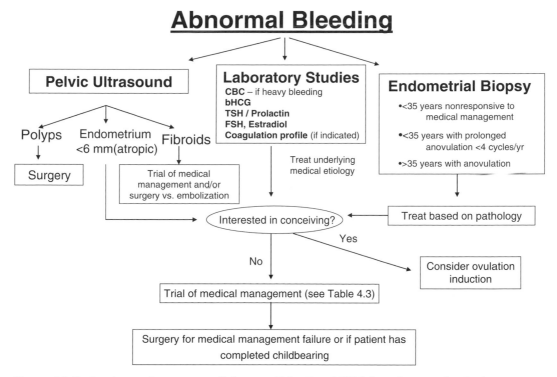

Figure 4.1 Evaluation and treatment of abnormal bleeding. bHCG, beta-human chorionic gonadotropin; CBC, complete blood count; FSH, follicle-stimulating hormone; TSH, thyrotropin-stimulating hormone.

low FSH is a functional ovarian cyst. Interpretation of FSH and estradiol testing is reviewed in Figure 4.2.

Endometrial biopsy

Endometrial sampling with an endometrial biopsy may be considered based on the degree of abnormal bleeding in patients, the patient's history, and her age. Endometrial biopsy is suggested for patients age 35 years or younger nonresponsive to medical therapy, those age 35 years or younger with prolonged periods of unopposed estrogen (e.g., PCOS), and those age 35 or older with suspected anovulatory bleeding.

After excluding pregnancy, an endometrial biopsy is performed by cleansing the cervix with an antiseptic solution and passing a 3 mm Pipelle (Cooper Surgical, Trumbull, CT, United States) through the cervix. The Pipelle is placed at the uterine fundus and gently rotated in order to obtain an adequate endometrial sample.

Endometrial biopsy is associated with an accuracy rate comparable to that seen with D&C and agrees with findings at the time of hysterectomy in approximately 95% of cases. Treatment will depend on the pathologic diagnosis. Hyperplasia without atypia is often managed with a D&C or progestin therapy with a repeat biopsy after 3–6 months. Further evaluation is warranted if the hyperplasia persists. Any finding of hyperplasia with atypia requires further counseling and treatment, including consideration of surgery.

Transvaginal sonography

TVS is the most helpful tool to evaluate anatomic causes of bleeding. TVS may reveal gross uterine pathology such as polyps, cancers, uterine fibroids, or adnexal pathology. The most frequent pathology found is uterine fibroids. These may vary in size and location. They have a characteristic sonographic appearance with variable echogenicity and acoustic shadows generated

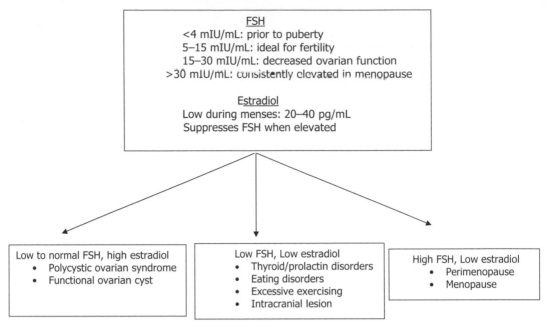

Figure 4.2 Utility of cycle day 2–3 testing of follicle-stimulating hormone (FSH) and estradiol.

by the dense fibroid tissue. They may contain echolucent cavities from central necrosis of the fibroid. TVS may suggest adenomyosis, but magnetic resonance imaging is superior to ultrasound in signifying the presence of adenomyosis, with a sensitivity of more than 80%.

TVS may also be used to detect any ovarian pathology that may be contributing to uterine bleeding. Although ultrasound is not practical to assess the event of ovulation, there are findings that may be visualized that indicate the probability of ovulatory cycles, such as the formation of an ovulatory follicle at midcycle (day 12–16) and a corpus luteum after ovulation. Other findings on TVS that may aid in determining the underlying etiology of bleeding include benign functional cysts, endometriomas, ovarian cancers, and polycystic ovaries.

Benign functional cysts are echolucent and thin walled with no nodularity of the cyst wall. They may vary in size from 20 to 30 mm but should be differentiated from an ovulatory follicle, which should only be present midcycle. If a simple-appearing cyst is visualized, the scan should be repeated during the early follicular phase (day 2–3) to assure that the structure was

not a midcycle ovulatory follicle. A corpus luteum cyst may also be seen in an ovulatory patient in the luteal phase of the cycle. A corpus luteum has a typical irregular increased echogenicity and is well delineated from the surrounding ovarian tissue; it has an appearance very similar to that of an endometrioma. The scan should be repeated in the early follicular phase if there is a suspicion of endometriosis as a corpus luteum should have regressed by this point. If the same cyst is present, there is an increased probability that an endometrioma is present.

Polycystic ovaries may also be seen with TVS. Multiple small (less than 10 mm) follicles crowded along the periphery of the ovary are visualized. Findings of polycystic ovaries aid in the diagnosis and are used as one of the diagnostic criteria of the syndrome. Pathologic large ovarian cysts and masses may also be visualized with TVS. Any ultrasonographic finding suspicious of a malignancy (irregular cyst walls, papillations, solid and cystic components) warrants further investigation.

The endometrium can also be evaluated during an TVS examination. The thickness and sonographic appearance of the normal endometrium vary during the menstrual cycle. Endometrial thickness is assessed in the midline sagittal plane and includes the full width of the endometrium including the anterior and posterior walls of the uterus. During menses, the endometrium is thin and not clearly delineated. In the proliferative phase, the endometrial stripe develops a multi-layered sonographic appearance; the wider inner portion of the proliferative endometrium is hypoechoic, and the outer portion is relatively hyperechoic. In the secretory phase, the endometrial stripe thickens to a mean of 10–16 mm in width and becomes diffusely hyperechoic secondary to accumulation of mucus and glycogen in the increasingly tortuous glands. In the absence of obvious anatomic pathology and with an endometrial thickness of less than 5 mm, there is unlikely to be any pathology present, and bleeding is likely due to anovulation or atrophy (menopausal).

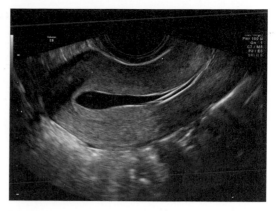

Figure 4.3 Normal intrauterine cavity on saline infusion sonography.

Saline infusion sonography

SIS (sonohysterography) enhances endovaginal ultrasound examination of the uterine cavity with minimal patient discomfort. SIS consists of using TVS to image the uterine cavity while sterile saline is instilled into the cavity. This allows detection of abnormalities within the uterine cavity. SIS is performed by first cleansing the cervix with an antiseptic solution. A small intrauterine insemination catheter purged of any air bubbles is inserted through the cervix into the uterine cavity. Sterile saline is flushed through the catheter as the uterus is scanned in the long axis and coronal planes. Water appears dark and tissue is light so that they are easily visualized. Figure 4.3 demonstrates a normal endometrial cavity on SIS. Uterine polyps (Figures 4.4 and 4.5), fibroids (Figures 4.6 and 4.7), and carcinomas will appear as focal filling defects in the uterine cavity.

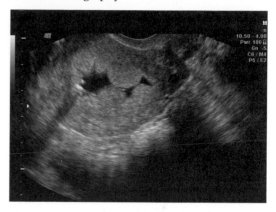

Figure 4.4 Endometrial polyps on saline infusion sonography (see also Figure 4.5).

The accuracy of SIS approximates hysteroscopy, but it is estimated that SIS may miss approximately 7% of intrauterine pathology that otherwise would have been detected by hysteroscopy. It is suggested that a thick endometrium may obscure small lesions in the cavity such as small endometrial polyps; therefore, SIS should be performed in the early follicular phase of the cycle after menses when the endometrium is

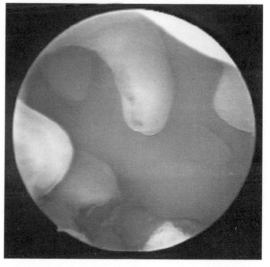

Figure 4.5 Endometrial polyps as visualized by hysteroscopy (see Plate 4.5).

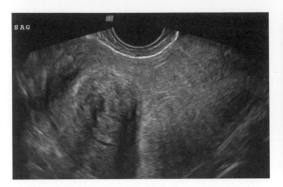

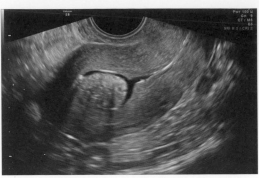

Figure 4.6 Fibroid visualized on transvaginal sonography.

Figure 4.7 A fibroid visualized with saline infusion sonography, demonstrating a significant intracavitary component.

thinnest. This also eliminates the concern over interrupting an early pregnancy that may be present in the luteal phase of the cycle. A pregnancy test should be performed prior to SIS if there is any possibility of pregnancy.

SIS is a safe procedure, but the risks include pelvic infection of 1% so it should not be performed if there is suspicion of an active uterine or vaginal infection. The procedure is generally very well tolerated but may cause mild cramping, spotting, and/or discharge.

Sterile saline is flushed through the catheter as the uterus is scanned in the long axis and coronal planes. Small filling defects are noted for size and location in the uterine cavity. Polyps may be seen originating from the endometrium, and fibroids may also be seen whether they are intracavitary or submucosal.

★ **TIPS & TRICKS**

Uterine filling defects within the cavity of the uterus are often difficult to detect as the echogenicity of polyps and fibroids is similar to that of the adjacent endometrium. Saline infusion sonography (SIS or sonohysterography) enhances endovaginal ultrasound examination and is one of the most useful tools in the evaluation of abnormal uterine bleeding. SIS is able to detect even small abnormalities in the endometrial cavity of the uterus that otherwise may not be able to be visualized with traditional ultrasound.

SIS can be performed easily with minimal patient discomfort. SIS is performed by first cleansing the cervix with an antiseptic solution. A small intrauterine insemination catheter purged of any air bubbles is inserted through the cervix into the uterine cavity.

Hysteroscopy

Hysteroscopy with direct visualization of the uterine cavity and biopsy of intrauterine abnormalities is considered the "gold standard" for the diagnosis of intracavitary pathology such as uterine polyps (Figure 4.5 above) and fibroids. Hysteroscopy may also avoid the need for more major surgery such as hysterectomy. Hysteroscopy utilizes distension media and a telescopic instrument that is inserted into the uterine cavity to directly visualize uterine abnormalities and allow access for the biopsy and/or resection of specific lesions. Hysteroscopy may be performed in an office or operating room setting. Generally, an operating room setting with access to adequate anesthesia is better tolerated and provides improved access to perform additional operative procedures when indicated. Pregnancy, genital tract infection, and uterine carcinoma are contraindications to hysteroscopy. Complications include hemorrhage, fluid embolization, perforation, visceral injury, infection, and fluid overload.

A variety of distending media may be used for adequate visualization of the uterine cavity. Carbon dioxide gas may be used and avoids the use of liquid, which contains air bubbles. However, the disadvantage is the risk of gas embolization, and it requires monitoring of intrauterine pressures. Most hysteroscopy is performed with liquid media. Different liquid media may be differentiated by their viscosity and electrolyte content. High-viscosity fluid (Dextran 70) is a thick liquid that provides excellent visibility during hysteroscopy. However, it has a higher risk of damaging the equipment over time if this not properly cleaned after the procedure, and it has a higher risk of vascular fluid overload since it is a plasma expander. Fluid volume should not exceed 500 mL, which is a significant disadvantage to the use of this agent. Given the concern over fluid overload, devices are available that monitor fluid inflow and outflow for assessment of overall fluid deficit. In addition, guidelines are available for fluid monitoring.

Low-viscosity fluids may be used as an alternative to high-viscosity agents. Low-viscosity fluids may contain electrolytes or be relatively low in electrolyte concentration. Low-electrolyte agents (glycine 1.5%, mannitol 5%, sorbitol 3%) are hyposmolar and can cause hyponatremia and subsequent cerebral edema if used in excess; therefore, the total amount of fluid deficit should not exceed 1,000 mL, and very close monitoring should be performed. The advantage of these agents is that they may be used with radiofrequency energy for cutting and desiccating tissue using monopolar energy. This is particularly helpful in the surgical treatment of polyps and fibroids, and for endometrial ablations.

Fortunately, it is possible to use electrolyte fluids that are low viscosity (normal saline, lactated Ringer's solution) with bipolar energy. These low-viscosity fluids have the disadvantage of decreased visibility if there is bleeding present in the uterine cavity. However, they have the significant advantage of being isotonic, and therefore the risk of hyponatremia is significantly decreased. Fluid overload and pulmonary edema is possible, so fluid balance should be monitored closely.

Treatment of abnormal bleeding

Treatment of irregular bleeding will depend on the severity of the bleeding and the underlying etiology. Severe acute bleeding in adults may be secondary to intrauterine pathology (typically fibroids or cancers) or a coagulopathy. Hormonal etiologies of bleeding typically do not frequently present with severe bleeding or hemodynamic instability. For patients with severe acute bleeding, the primary treatment goal is to stabilize the patient. An investigation into the etiology may be undertaken expediently while the patient is being stabilized with medical management (Table 4.3).

Fortunately, most bleeding is not severe and can be managed medically. Generally, medical management is attempted prior to surgery and will depend on the specific etiology and the patient's desire for either pregnancy or contraception. Further fertility evaluation and ovulation induction may be needed to regulate menstrual cycles to achieve pregnancy. Menstrual irregularities may be treated with a variety of medical management options for patients desiring contraception and/or not currently interested in achieving pregnancy.

Table 4.3 Hormonal management of uterine bleeding

Combination oral contraceptive pills
30–35 mg monophasic pill cyclically, with withdrawal bleeding periodically (every 3 months) or continuously
• Breakthrough bleeding is common, with long durations between withdrawal bleeds, but by 1 year most patients will be amenorrheic • For severe acute bleeding, prescribe up to four times daily dosing for 1–4 days; then taper to three times a day for 3 days, and then twice daily for 2 days, before giving daily to cycle • Alternatives for patients who prefer a nonoral administration include transdermal or a vaginal ring, but dosing cannot be adjusted with these routes

Table 4.3 *Continued*

Estrogens
Oral
Conjugated equine estrogen (1.25–2.5 mg)
Estradiol (1–2 mg)
• For severe acute bleeding, can use up to four doses in 24 hours and then switch to oral contraceptives • Dilatation and curettage after 2–4 doses if there is no response • May need to prescribe antiemetics for nausea secondary to high-dose estrogen side effects
Intravenous
Conjugated equine estrogen 25 mg intravenously every 4 hours for 24 hours
• Prescribed for severe acute bleeding with hospital admission • No definitive evidence that intravenous are superior to oral estrogens if the patient is able to tolerate oral administration • Start oral doses of oral contraceptives during intravenous treatment up to four times daily for 1–4 days; then taper to three times a day for 3 days, and then twice daily for 2 days, before giving daily to cycle
Progestins
Oral (given monthly for 14 days for cyclic withdrawal bleeds or may be given continuously)
Medroxyprogesterone acetate (10–20 mg)
Micronized progesterone (200 mg)
Norethindrone (0.35 mg)
• If given cyclically, it will not provide effective contraception • Best used for patients with polycystic ovarian syndrome or contraindications to estrogen • Often given continuously for the treatment of endometrial hyperplasia
Intramuscular
Depot medroxyprogesterone acetate (Depo-Provera 150 mg intramuscularly every 3 months)
• Irregular bleeding is common for several months, but many patients will become amenorrheic by 12 months
Implant
Implanon (etonogestrel administered in a 3-year implant)
• Irregular bleeding is common for several months, but many patients will become amenorrheic by 12 months
Intrauterine device
Mirena (levonorgestrel administered via a 5-year intrauterine device)
• Irregular bleeding is common for several months, but many patients will become amenorrheic by 12 months

*Consider the addition of nonsteroidal anti-inflammatory agents to hormonal treatment for control of abnormal uterine bleeding.

Medical management

Medical management of abnormal bleeding will depend on the underlying etiology. Anatomic causes of abnormal bleeding are most effectively treated with surgery; however, a trial of medical management is often appropriate for stable patients prior to consideration of surgery. Anovulatory bleeding is best treated hormonally. There are a variety of medical management options available, and treatment should be tailored to the patient considering the underlying etiology of her bleeding as well as her desire for pregnancy, need for contraception, preference, and contraindications to treatment. Medical treatment options include prostaglandin synthetase inhibitors, antifibrinolytics, oral contraceptive pills, and other hormones. The most commonly used hormonal options are summarized in Table 4.3.

Nonhormonal agents

Nonsteroidal anti-inflammatory drugs
Prostaglandins, prostacyclin (PGI2), and thromboxane A2 are important in endometrial hemostasis by affecting the balance of vasoconstriction/vasodilatation and platelet aggregation. The prostaglandins PGE2 and PGF2-alpha increase during the menstrual cycle and are found in menstrual effluent. Nonsteroidal anti-inflammatory drugs (NSAIDs) inhibit prostaglandin synthesis and decrease menstrual blood loss. NSAIDs also alter the balance of thromboxane A2 and prostacyclin, allowing for further regulation of bleeding. Several NSAIDs are available, including ibuprofen, naproxen, and mefenamic acid. They should be initiated prior to the onset of bleeding for maximum effectiveness and have the added benefit of reducing menstrual cramping. They have been found to reduce menstrual blood loss by approximately 30%. The primary concern over the long-term use of NSAIDs is the risk of gastrointestinal bleeding and ulcers. Their use is contraindicated in patients with allergies to acetylsalicylic acid (aspirin) and in those with gastrointestinal ulcers or reactive pulmonary disease.

Antifibrinolytics
Tranexamic acid is an over-the-counter antifibrinolytic agent used primarily in Europe for the control of bleeding. It is a synthetic form of the amino acid lysine. It is used in the United States for control of bleeding during surgery for patients with hemophilia. The dose is 25 mg/kg 3–4 times a day beginning 1 day prior to surgery. It has been considered as a treatment for menorrhagia due to the fact that it has been shown to decrease the amount of menstrual bleeding through its hemostatic mechanism. Side effects include headache, nausea, and gastrointestinal distress. There is some concern that this agent may increase the risk of blood clots so patients with risk factors should consider avoiding this agent.

Agents used for patients with bleeding disorders
The etiology of bleeding in patients with bleeding disorders is decreased blood clotting. Desmopressin stimulates the release of blood factors that are helpful in patients with bleeding disorders such as von Willebrand disease. Desmopressin has been shown to reduce menorrhagia in women with von Willebrand disease and mild hemophilia. Side effects include headache, nausea, and weakness. Its use has not been studied extensively in women with menorrhagia that is not secondary to a bleeding disorder; therefore, its use is not justified.

Hormonal agents

Combination oral contraceptives
Combined oral contraceptives are generally the mainstay of treatment for abnormal uterine bleeding and are effective for contraception. They reduce menstrual blood loss by 50% in women with bleeding secondary to ovulatory or anovulatory causes. Oral contraceptives contain a combination of estrogen and a progestin and reduce menstrual blood loss through a variety of mechanisms including inhibiting ovulation and inducing endometrial decidualization and atrophy. Oral contraceptives may be taken cyclically or continuously and are categorized as monophasic, biphasic, or triphasic. Both biphasic and triphasic regimens vary the amount of hormone throughout the pill cycle. There is a paucity of data directly comparing the effectiveness of these regimens for control of irregular and/or heavy bleeding compared to monophasic regimens. In addition, they are difficult to compare as the type of progestin differs between them. In fact, however, the monophasic regimen

is often recommended due to its consistent hormonal profile.

Oral contraceptives may be prescribed to non-smoking perimenopausal patients who have no contraindications or risk factors (see Caution box). There are other methods for delivery of combination estrogen and progestin such as patches and vaginal rings. However, it is not known if there is any advantage or disadvantage for patients with irregular menstrual bleeding. One disadvantage to nonoral routes is that dosing cannot be easily adjusted.

✋ CAUTION

Although oral contraceptive pills are used commonly to treat a variety of types of abnormal uterine bleeding, there are several contraindications, including migraine headaches with focal neurologic symptoms, age greater than 35 years and a cigarette smoker, and a history of thromboembolic disease, coronary artery disease, congestive heart failure, cerebrovascular disease, hypertension with vascular disease or older than 35 years, diabetes with vascular disease or older than 35 years, systemic lupus erythematosus with vascular disease, nephritis, or antiphospholipid antibodies and hypertriglyceridemia. Alternative forms of medical or surgical management should be considered in patients with these contraindications.

Estrogens

Estrogen therapy is most helpful for endometrial bleeding secondary to an atrophic endometrium. Estrogen is required to stimulate the growth of endometrial tissue from the basal layer of the endometrium. It is helpful for estrogen breakthrough bleeding in patients with low estradiol levels (perimenopausal) or hypogonadotropic patients. It is often helpful after heavy prolonged bleeding to stabilize the denuded endometrium. When bleeding is acute and heavy, high-dose estrogen therapy is indicated (Table 4.3).

Estrogen is also helpful for bleeding attributed to progesterone breakthrough, as found in patients treated with oral contraceptives or progestin-only treatments. Over time, the endometrium becomes atrophic in response to progestin and requires estrogen for stabilization. It is important to remember that the contraindications for oral contraceptives also apply to the use of systemic estrogen therapy.

Progestins

Progestins have traditionally been reserved for patients that have contraindications to estrogen or clearly have bleeding caused by unopposed estrogen (e.g., PCOS). They have the advantages of reducing bleeding and protecting against uterine cancer. Progestins are either natural progestin (progesterone) or synthetic (medroxyprogesterone, norethindrone acetate, norgestrel), and come in several different delivery systems (oral, intramuscular, IUD, implantable) Oral forms may be prescribed continuously, but they often are prescribed in a cyclic regimen for 10–14 days each cycle to induce withdrawal bleeding. It is important to remember that cyclic progestins are not effective for pregnancy prevention as they do not prevent ovulation effectively if given for only 10–14 days each cycle. Progestins are contraindicated in patients with breast cancer, unexplained abnormal vaginal bleeding, or pregnancy. The side effects of all progestins include irregular breakthrough bleeding, bloating, depression, and mood swings. The injectable form also may result in prolonged amenorrhea for several months after the last injection.

There are several routes of administration for progestins for patients that would prefer a nonoral route or desire more effective contraception. Continuous routes include the implant (Implanon), IUD (Mirena), and injectable (Depo-Provera). Depo-Provera is medroxyprogesterone acetate that is injected every 3 months. Implanon is an implantable form of progestin containing the active ingredient etonogestrel. It is approved for 3 years of use and continuously releases progestin. These delivery methods are effective for contraception as the continuous administration results in endometrial decidualization and atrophy. The side effects are similar to other forms of progestin, but the primary side effect is breakthrough bleeding.

Progestin may also be delivered in the form of a levonorgestrel-releasing IUD (Mirena).

Levonorgestrel is derived from 19-nortestosterone and suppresses endometrial development. The progestin acts locally at the endometrium and cervix and has few systemic hormonal effects compared to oral, injectable, or implant administration. It is effective for contraception, with failure rates similar to Depo-Provera and Implanon of less than 1%. A recent systematic review concluded that this IUD appears equally as effective as hysterectomy in improving quality of life. The IUD has also been shown in some studies to reduce menstrual blood loss in patients with adenomyosis, endometriosis, and fibroid-related menorrhagia, but further studies are needed. The IUD requires changing every 5 years. The complications include expulsion (1 in 20), cramping (particularly at insertion), perforation at insertion (1 in 1000), and infection (1 in 100).

Danazol

Danazol is a synthetic androgen that suppresses LH and FSH, resulting in estrogen deprivation. The suppression of estrogen and subsequent endometrial atrophy results in decreased uterine bleeding. Unfortunately, its side effects have limited its use. Adverse side effects include hirsutism, acne, weight gain, and deepening of the voice. It may also adversely impact lipoprotein profiles. Pregnant women or those attempting pregnancy must also avoid this medication due to the risk of birth defects and masculinization of a female fetus. Due to these concerns, danazol is not used as a first-line agent for control of menorrhagia.

Gonadotropin-releasing hormone agonists and antagonists

GnRH agonists and antagonists block the release of LH and FSH from the pituitary. This results in suppression of ovulation, and endometrial atrophy secondary to suppression of estrogen. They are not indicated for long-term use due to the significant suppression of estrogen and the subsequent risk of osteopenia and osteoporosis. Their use is typically limited to 6 months and is reserved for patients in preparation for surgery (prior to hysterectomy, myomectomy, or endometrial ablation) or patients with chronic medical conditions (e.g., renal disease, coagu-

lopathies) that require significant endometrial suppression.

Surgical management

Approximately 60% of women are unsatisfied with medical treatment and pursue surgical intervention within 2 years of medical management. Surgical management may be considered when medical management of bleeding fails or contraindications exist against medical management. A D&C is rarely therapeutic for long-term management; it is best used for the acute treatment of severe bleeding or as a diagnostic procedure to obtain a sample of the endometrium for pathologic evaluation. A better alternative combines hysteroscopy and D&C to directly visualize the endometrial cavity and evaluate for specific organic lesions. Using this combined approach, endometrial polyps and submucous uterine leiomyomas may be identified and resected hysteroscopically. Additional surgical treatment options include endometrial ablation and hysterectomy.

Hysteroscopy

Hysteroscopy may be utilized for both diagnostic and therapeutic purposes. Diagnostic hysteroscopy may visualize pathology to determine a diagnosis. Operative hysteroscopy may be performed to resect those abnormalities such as polyps or fibroids under direct visualization. A variety of distending agents are available as discussed previously, and the choice of medium will depend on the surgeon's preference and the equipment used to resect these abnormalities. Hysteroscopic resection of lesions is relatively noninvasive, with less morbidity than hysterectomy, and allows a patient to retain her uterus for future childbearing.

Endometrial ablation

Endometrial ablation may be considered in women who have completed childbearing as long as hyperplasia and cancer have been excluded. Endometrial ablation destroys the endometrium to control menorrhagia. The majority of patients have an improvement in bleeding or complete amenorrhea, but there is an approximately 0–15% failure rate. Endometrial ablation is most effective if performed when the endometrium is thin. This can be assured by scheduling the procedure after menses or hormonal therapy to induce endometrial atrophy. There are many modalities for endometrial ablation. Traditional methods of endometrial ablation involved hysteroscopy and laser ablation of the endometrium, rollerball desiccation, or resection of the endometrium with a loop. Advantages include direct visualization of the endometrium during the procedure, but disadvantages include those of hysteroscopy, including fluid overload. Newer methods for ablating the endometrium without necessitating hysteroscopy have been developed.

One technique involves utilizing an intrauterine balloon that uniformly distributes heated fluid that causes endometrial tissue necrosis (Thermachoice [Gynecare, Somerville, NJ, United States] and Cavaterm [Wallsten Medical SA, Morges, Switzerland]). Hydrothermal ablation (Hydro Therm-Ablator TM; BEI Medical Systems, Teterboro, NJ, United States) is another procedure used to perform endometrial ablation. With this technique, water fills the entire endometrial surface. Therefore, even significantly deformed uterine cavities that may not be amenable to the intrauterine balloon may be treated with this modality. The disadvantages of this technique include burns to the cervix or vagina, as well as the concern of burns to the peritoneal cavity.

Other techniques for endometrial ablation include the use of either bipolar desiccation (NovaSure; Novacept, Mountain View, CA, United States) or microwave ablation (FemWave; Microsulis, Waterlooville, Hampshire, United Kingdom). Bipolar desiccation is performed by insertion of a disposable expandable mesh that is placed into the uterine cavity and expands to the shape of the cavity. Microwave ablation is performed by placing the active tip of the device into the cavity, microwave energy being swept through the cavity to desiccate the tissue.

Overall, endometrial ablation has several appealing advantages over hysterectomy. The operative time and complication rate are significantly decreased, but there is a risk of persistent or recurrent bleeding and future repeat surgery. However, there does not seem to be a significant difference between the different types of endometrial ablation. Most of the newer techniques are technically easier than hysteroscopy-based methods, and the success rates and complication profiles compare favorably.

Alternative interventions

There are several nonsurgical alternatives to treat uterine fibroids. Uterine artery embolization (UAE) may be the best treatment option for women with symptomatic fibroids who are not candidates for surgery or who do not wish to accept the risks of an operative procedure. UAE is an outpatient procedure performed by catheterizing the femoral artery and through this approach isolating the uterine artery to deliver particulate material to the vessels supplying the fibroid. The material occludes the vessels, which results in ischemic necrosis of the fibroid. The procedure is most effective for patients with a single fibroid but may be considered for patients with additional fibroids. Pregnancy, active infection, and suspicion of uterine or ovarian cancer are absolute contraindications to UAE. Relative contraindications include coagulopathy, immunocompromise, prior pelvic irradiation, a desire to maintain childbearing potential, contrast allergy, and large, pedunculated, or subserosal myomas.

Hysterectomy

Hysterectomy may be considered if other modalities fail or if organic pathology (e.g., significant uterine leiomyomas, carcinoma) preclude the use of more conservative surgery. Hysterectomy may be considered instead of more conservative surgery such as hysteroscopy or endometrial ablation for patients who prefer definitive treatment and/or have completed childbearing.

EVIDENCE AT A GLANCE

Results from meta-analyses show the following:
* There is a significant decrease in blood loss for patients treated with oral contraceptives, nonsteroidal anti-inflammatory drugs, or danazol. However, there is little evidence that one treatment is most effective.
* Cyclic progestin therapy is significantly less effective at reducing menstrual blood

loss when compared with tranexamic acid, danazol, and the progesterone-releasing intrauterine system.

- Surgery, especially hysterectomy, reduces menstrual bleeding at 1 year more than medical treatments, but the progestin intrauterine device appears equally effective in improving quality of life.

Summary

Menstrual disorders are common during the reproductive years and require appropriate evaluation and treatment. Evaluation includes testing for both anatomic and hormonal causes of bleeding, which may be pathologic or physiologic. A variety of medical and surgical treatment options is available depending on the underlying etiology. Treatment should be tailored to the patient, considering her desire for pregnancy, her need for contraception, her preference, and any contraindications to treatment.

Selected bibliography

American College of Obstetricians and Gynecologists. ACOG Technology Assessment in Obstetrics and Gynecology, number 4, hysteroscopy. Obstet Gynecol 2005;106: 439–42.

American College of Obstetrics and Gynecology. Management of anovulatory bleeding. Practice Bulletin No. 14. In: ACOG Compendium of selected publications. Washington, DC: ACOG: 2000. Available from: http://www.acog.org/publications/educational_bulletins/pb014.cfm.

American College of Obstetrics and Gynecology. Practice Bulletin. The use of hormonal contraception in women with coexisting medical conditions. In: ACOG Compendium of selected publications. Washington, DC: ACOG: 2002. p. 503.

deKroon CD, deBock GH, Diehen SW, Jansen FW. Saline contract hysterosonography in abnormal uterine bleeding: a systematic review and meta-analysis. Br J Obstet Gynecol 2003;110: 938–47.

Ely JW, Kennedy CM, Clark EC, Bowdler NC. Abnormal uterine bleeding: a management algorithm. J Am Board Fam Med 2006;19: 590–602.

European Society of Human Reproduction and Embryology Capri Workshop Group. Endometrial bleeding. Human Repro Update 2007; 13:421–31.

Farquhar C, Brown J. Oral contraceptive pill for heavy menstrual bleeding. Cochrane Database of Sys Rev 2009, Issue 4. Art. No.: CD000154.

Filley RA. Ultrasound evaluation during the first trimester. In: Callen PW, ed. Ultrasonography in obstetrics and gynecology, 3rd edn. Philadelphia: WB Saunders; 1998. pp. 63–85.

Lethaby A, Hickey M, Garry R, Penninx J. Endometrial resection/ablation techniques for heavy menstrual bleeding. Cochrane Database Syst Rev 2009; Issue 4. Art. No.: CD001501.

Lethaby A, Irvine GA, Cameron IT. Cyclical progestogens for heavy menstrual bleeding. Cochrane Database of Sys Rev 2008, Issue 1. Art. No.: CD001016.

Loffer FD, Bradley LD, Brill AI, Brooks PG, Cooper JM. Hysteroscopic fluid monitoring guidelines. The ad hoc committee on hysteroscopic training guidelines of the American Association of Gynecologic Laparoscopists. J Am Assoc Gyn Laparosc 2000;7:167–8.

Marjoribanks J, Lethaby A, Farquhar C. Surgery versus medical therapy for heavy menstrual bleeding. Cochrane Database Syst Rev 2006, Issue 2. Art. No.: CD003855.

Phillip CS, Faiz A, Dowling NF et al. Development of a screening tool for identifying women with menorrhagia for hemostatic evaluation. Am J Obstet Gynec 2008;198:163e1–163e8.

Rotterdam ESHRE/ASRM-sponsored PCOS Consensus Workshop Group. Revised 2003 consensus on diagnostic criteria and long term health risks related to polycystic ovary syndrome. Fertil Steril 2004;81:19–23.

Salamonsen LA. Tissue injury and repair in the female human reproductive tract. Reproduction 2003;125:301.

5

Abnormal Menstrual Bleeding in Hyperandrogenic Ovulatory Dysfunction

Rebecca S. Usadi

Carolinas Medical Center, Charlotte, North Carolina, USA

Introduction

Hyperandrogenic ovulatory dysfunction, commonly called polycystic ovarian syndrome or PCOS, is the most common endocrine disorder of reproductive-aged women. Women with this condition are prone to a variety of abnormal types of menstrual bleeding as well as metabolic and endocrine disorders. This chapter will review the common clinical presentations, etiology, and diagnostic evaluation of hyperandrogenic ovulatory disorders. A discussion of treatment will highlight therapies directed at improving the menstrual function and medical and reproductive condition of women with PCOS.

Pathophysiology of polycystic ovarian syndrome

Epidemiology and genetic basis of the syndrome

The best estimates report PCOS as affecting 6–8% of women. The prevalence of this syndrome appears to be similar in varying ethnic backgrounds and geographic locations. One study showed a prevalence of approximately7% in the Southeast United States, the Greek isle of Lesbos, and Italy. The condition is a heterogeneous disorder and manifests differently in different ethnic and racial groups. For instance, South Asian women in the United Kingdom with PCOS have greater symptoms of hyperandrogenism, such as

hirsutism and acne, than Caucasians in the United Kingdom. American women with PCOS tend to have a higher body mass index (BMI) compared to Italian women with PCOS, and Mexican-American women with PCOS have higher rates of insulin resistance than Caucasian American women with PCOS.

There appears to be a strong hereditary component to the disorder, with the siblings and mothers of women with PCOS demonstrating sonographic evidence of the condition. The first large family study of PCOS in 1968 showed a high prevalence of oligomenorrhea in first-degree relatives of women diagnosed with PCOS based on ovarian wedge resection or culdoscopy. Many of the family studies since then have described an autosomal dominant inheritance. The clinical heterogeneity may be a reflection of the genetic heterogeneity of the syndrome. Multiple genetic markers have been investigated as causative factors in PCOS. Altered genetic expression in PCOS affects pathways regulating steroidogenesis, gonadotropin and steroid hormone function, insulin action and secretion, and metabolic action. The underlying genetic dysfunction may vary in differing populations.

Androgen secretion in women with polycystic ovarian syndrome

Androgens are produced in the ovaries, the adrenal glands, and the periphery (mostly the

Disorders of Menstruation, 1st edition. Edited by Paul B. Marshburn and Bradley S. Hurst.
© 2011 Blackwell Publishing Ltd.

skin). The ovary secretes mostly testosterone and androstenedione. The adrenal glands secrete about the same amount of androstenedione as the ovary. The adrenal glands are almost exclusively responsible for secretion of dehydroepiandrosterone (DHEAS) and secrete very little testosterone. Therefore, testosterone is the primary marker of ovarian androgen production, and DHEAS is the primary marker of adrenal androgen production.

High insulin levels also reduce SHBG concentrations. All of these factors lead to the decreased SHBG concentration in women with PCOS and the increased concentration of free serum testosterone.

Interestingly, not all women with PCOS always have elevated serum androgen levels as there is a range of individual variability. That is why the diagnostic criteria include both clinical symptoms and biochemical levels of hyperandrogenism.

Etiology of PCOS

The endocrine etiology of PCOS is quite complex and remains a topic of great discussion. There is a clear aberrant neuroendocrine pathway involved with persistently rapid secretion of gonadotropin-releasing hormone (GnRH). The abnormal secretion of GnRH, in turn, stimulates chronically elevated luteinizing hormone (LH) release from the pituitary, which drives the testosterone production from the ovary. The PCOS ovary itself demonstrates altered testosterone secretion from its theca cells in culture in response to LH stimulation. Hyperinsulinemia also drives androgen secretion by direct action on insulin receptors on the ovary and indirectly by affecting sex hormone-binding globulin (SHBG) and insulin-like growth factor-1 (Figure 5.1). The pediatric and adolescent endocrine literature reveal that elevated insulin levels often predate the development of elevated androgen levels.

Clinical presentation

Hyperandrogenism in women often presents with a combination of dermatologic and gynecologic symptoms. Hirsutism and acne are the most common dermatologic manifestations of hyperandrogenism. Other skin disorders may develop, including seborrhea, alopecia, and acanthosis nigricans. Elevated androgen levels often manifest with ovulatory dysfunction and subsequent menstrual irregularities and infertility. These women are also at risk for other endocrine and metabolic disorders such as obesity, insulin resistance, hypertension, and lipid disorders.

⚛ SCIENCE REVISITED

The peripheral action of the enzyme 5-alpha reductase converts testosterone into dihydrotestosterone (DHT). DHT is responsible for the effect of androgens on the skin and external genitalia. Testosterone and DHT are the most bioactive androgens. Measurement of serum DHT, however, is difficult due to its high turnover and affinity for sex hormone-binding globulin (SHBG). Serum 3-alpha androstenediol glucuronide (3α diolG), a metabolite of DHT, serves as a better marker of androgen action in the periphery. 3α diolG, however, is not commonly used in clinical practice as a marker of hyperandrogenism as it does not serve to change any clinical diagnosis or treatment beyond what can be assessed clinically (i.e., degree of hirsutism or Ferriman–Gallwey scoring).

Both ovarian and adrenal androgen concentrations are elevated in women with polycystic ovarian syndrome (PCOS). The biologic activity of testosterone is mostly determined by SHBG binding. Free or unbound testosterone is the most potent biologic form of androgen. Women with PCOS tend to have low SHBG levels. Low SHBG levels allow a higher concentration of testosterone to remain in the unbound form, resulting in symptoms of hyperandrogenism. SHBG concentration is decreased in the setting of obesity and high androgen levels, and increased in the setting of high estradiol levels. In fact, body mass index is positively correlated with serum testosterone levels and inversely correlated with serum SHBG levels.

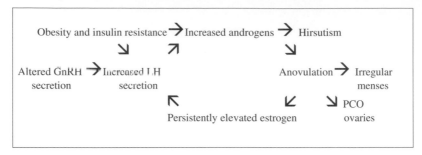

Figure 5.1 Pathophysiology of polycystic ovarian (PCO) syndrome. GnRH, gonadotrophin-releasing hormone; LH, luteinizing hormone.

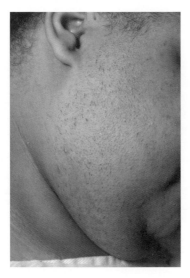

Figure 5.2 Facial hirsutism (see Plate 5.2).

Dermatologic manifestations

About 60% of hyperandrogenic women demonstrate hirsutism, typically beginning at menarche and progressing with age or weight gain. It is important to differentiate hirsutism from virilization or hypertrichosis. Hirsutism is described as the presence of hair in locations where women typically do not grow hair. It refers specifically to androgen-dependent hair growth mostly in the midline distribution. This includes facial hair on the upper lip, sideburns, and chin (Figure 5.2), chest hair and back hair. Androgen-sensitive areas on the lower body include a male pattern pubic hair distribution with increased hair on the inner thighs and buttocks.

Virilization is caused by excessive levels of androgen secretion and masculinization, and may be caused by androgen-secreting tumors or adrenal hyperplasia. Signs of virilization include voice deepening, temporal balding, clitoromegaly, and increased muscle mass. Hypertrichosis is excess vellus hair growth in nonandrogen-dependent areas, such as the arms. Medical conditions associated with hypertrichosis include anorexia nervosa, malnutrition, porphyria, and hypothyroidism. Several medications have been associated with hypertrichosis, such as minoxidil, phenytoin, and cyclosporine. An easy way to distinguish hirsutism from hypertrichosis is by using a Ferriman–Gallwey chart. The Ferriman–Gallwey score assigns a point score to the nine androgen-sensitive areas of hair growth. A score of 8 or greater is consistent with hyperandrogenism (Figure 5.3). One word of caution advised when using this scoring system is that it was developed using Caucasian subjects and may not be applicable to all ethnicities.

Acne is present in about a third of women with PCOS. It primarily affects the face but may be present on the back or chest as well. There is no clear correlation between androgen levels and severity of acne. Androgenic alopecia is a less common manifestation of PCOS, reported in about 10% of women with PCOS. Alopecia in women with PCOS typically begins with diffuse hair loss over the crown with a widening of the hair part.

Acanthosis nigricans and skin tags are other dermatologic conditions commonly present in women with PCOS. Acanthosis nigricans is the presence of dark, velvety, thickened skin found in the skin folds of the posterior neck, the axillae, under the breasts, and the groins (Figure 5.4). Acanthosis is highly associated with the hyperin-

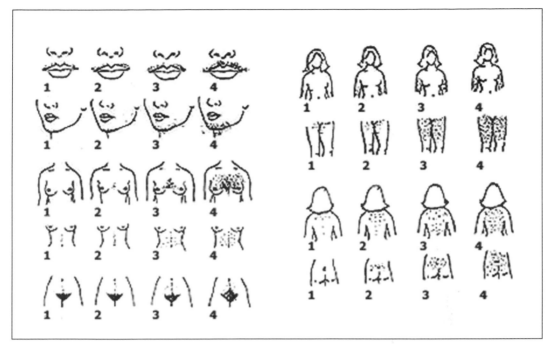

Figure 5.3 Ferriman–Gallwey chart. Reproduced with permission from Elsevier. The figure was published in Hatch, R, Rosenfield, RS, Kim, MH, Tredway, D. Hirsutism: implications, etiology, and management. Am J Obstet Gynecol 1981;140:815. Copyright Elsevier 1981.

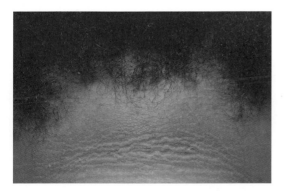

Figure 5.4 Acanthosis nigricans (see Plate 5.4).

sulinemic state of PCOS. The exact etiology is unknown but is thought to be an increased action of growth factors, such as insulin-like growth factor, on the keratinocytes and fibroblasts in the skin. Acanthosis is often considered a reliable marker of hyperinsulinemia, glucose intolerance, and frank diabetes.

Menstrual and reproductive abnormalities in hyperandrogenic women

PCOS is one of the most common causes of menstrual irregularities; it can present with amenorrhea and dysfunctional uterine bleeding. Approximately 80% of women with PCOS experience oligomenorrhea. About 2% of women with hyperandrogenic ovulatory dysfunction experience polymenorrhea characterized by frequent menses less than 26 days apart. Often oligomenorrhea is punctuated by episodes of menorrhagia and sometimes by acute vaginal bleeding. In a hyperandrogenic woman, the underlying etiology is most often anovulatory bleeding. These women are in a state of chronic unopposed estrogen and do not undergo regular endogenous progesterone withdrawal bleeding. The presence of obesity in many of these women further exacerbates the state of unopposed estrogen due to the increasing circulating levels of estrone, a weak estrogen secreted from adipose tissue. Chronic estrogen exposure leads to a thickening of the endometrium with irregular, unpredictable shedding and bleeding. One retrospective cohort study reported an incidence of hysterectomy three times higher in women with POCS than controls for benign indications of dysfunctional bleeding.

Typically, the symptoms of PCOS begin with the onset of puberty. The diagnosis of PCOS in adolescents cannot be made on the basis of oligomenorrhea alone as many adolescents experience anovulatory cycles for the first few years after menarche. The diagnosis of PCOS in adolescents therefore requires the presence of hyperandrogenism along with the ovulatory dysfunction or polycystic-appearing ovaries, just as in adult women. There appears to be an increased risk of PCOS in girls who develop premature pubarche. PCOS and menstrual abnormalities typically develop in women during episodes of weight gain, and puberty is a time when girls often gain some weight. Often women have a history of regular menstrual cycles but later develop PCOS and menstrual irregularities after a period of weight gain in later adult life. One scenario is a woman who has had normal menses but develops oligomenorrhea and PCOS symptoms after pregnancy weight gain.

Ovulatory dysfunction is the leading cause of infertility in women with PCOS. PCOS also effects fecundity even when treatment with ovulation induction or in-vitro fertilization (IVF) is administered. Live birth rates are lower in obese women with PCOS compared to lean women with PCOS. Both PCOS and obesity are independent risks for infertility and lower fecundity rates even with fertility treatment.

Endocrine and metabolic consequences of polycystic ovarian syndrome

Approximately 50% of women with PCOS are obese. The prevalence of obesity in women with PCOS varies by country. For instance, there is a higher prevalence of overweight and obese women with PCOS in the United States compared to women with PCOS in many European countries. The distribution of body fat in women with PCOS is different than the distribution of body fat in obese women without PCOS. Women with PCOS tend to have high concentrations of central and visceral adipose. Central

and visceral adipose is more metabolically active, predisposing them to an increased prevalence of insulin resistance and increased long-term risk of cardiovascular disease. Obesity therefore plays a central role in the pathophysiology of PCOS, by reducing SHBG, increasing androgens, and increasing the risk of insulin resistance.

Insulin resistance is a common feature of PCOS. It is also common in the setting of obesity even in the absence of PCOS so it is not considered one of the diagnostic criteria. Insulin resistance is present in about 50–70% of women with PCOS. It is more common in the overweight and obese women with PCOS than in lean women with PCOS. Almost 60% of obese women with PCOS are hyperinsulinemic. There are several types of syndrome involving insulin resistance, some congenital and some acquired. There is some controversy over whether the classically described hyperandrogenic–insulin resistant–acanthosis nigricans (HAIR-AN) syndrome is a truly separate disorder from PCOS or actually represents a subset of PCOS accompanied by severe metabolic derangements including hyperinsulinemia.

⚗ SCIENCE REVISITED

There is a large body of literature suggesting that the underlying mechanism of hyperinsulinemia is defective phosphorylation of the insulin receptor, which leads to impaired insulin signaling. Other suggested mechanisms include decreased target tissue sensitivity, increased hepatic sensitivity, and impaired pancreatic beta-cell function.

These altered responses to insulin sensitivity are responsible for the increased prevalence of glucose intolerance and type 2 diabetes in this population. One large prospective study reported the prevalence of glucose intolerance as approximately 30% and of diabetes as 8% in women with PCOS. This study showed the prevalence of glucose intolerance to be almost three times higher in overweight women with PCOS compared to controls. These altered responses to insulin sensitivity also put women with PCOS at a significantly higher risk of developing gestational diabetes during their pregnancies.

Hyperinsulinemia associated with polycystic ovarian syndrome (PCOS) increases the risks of cardiovascular disease. Dyslipidemias are more common in women with PCOS. These women are at increased risk of having elevated triglyceride levels, low high-density lipoprotein cholesterol concentrations, and increased levels of atherogenic small, dense, low-density lipoprotein particles. Women with PCOS are also are greater risk of hypertension. These factors lead to the increased risk of atherogenic disease as noted by increased endothelial dysfunction, carotid artery intima media thickness, and coronary artery calcification noted in women with PCOS compared to controls. All of these conditions associated with PCOS (obesity, hyperinsulinemia, atherogenic dyslipidemias) confer a longer-term risk of cardiovascular events similar to that of metabolic syndrome.

There is some conflict in the medical literature regarding the medical consequences of PCOS in women of normal body weight. Most studies show that about 25% of lean women with PCOS have decreased insulin sensitivity. Some studies show altered markers of cardiovascular and diabetic risk in all women with PCOS, whereas others show that weight is the primary determinant. Adiponectin, a marker associated with insulin resistance, is decreased in women with PCOS independent of BMI. Highly sensitive C-reactive protein, a marker of vascular inflammation, is not increased in women with a normal BMI with PCOS.

Other medical conditions associated with PCOS

Obstructive sleep apnea, a disorder most common in overweight men, is more prevalent in women with PCOS compared to age- and weight-matched controls. It is thought that the combination of obesity and elevated androgen levels may predispose women with PCOS to an increased risk of sleep apnea.

There is also an increased prevalence of mood disorders, such as depression and anxiety, in women with PCOS. PCOS appears to be an independent risk factor for these psychiatric disorders, independent from obesity and infertility. Quality of life scores are lower in women with PCOS, who self-report lower self-esteem, decreased sexual satisfaction, and less social interaction than their peers.

Pregnancy-related risks of polycystic ovarian syndrome

Women with PCOS have almost twice the risk of having an adverse obstetric or neonatal outcome. Compared to women without PCOS, there is a greater risk of first-trimester miscarriage, pregnancy-induced hypertension, gestational diabetes, pre-eclampsia, antepartum hemorrhage, and operative delivery. The risk of first-trimester miscarriage is thought to be related to the elevated insulin, LH, and plasminogen activator inhibitor levels. The rate of first-trimester miscarriage has been reported to be 20–40% higher in women with PCOS than the general population. One study reported an incidence of first-trimester loss as high as 73% in women with PCOS. All of the obstetric risks appear to be greatest in women with PCOS with clinical hyperandrogenism and impaired insulin sensitivity. The main adverse neonatal outcome has been related to birth weight. There is an increased risk of both large and small for gestational age babies in women with PCOS.

There is an independent risk for miscarriage in women with PCOS who are obese as well. Compared to lean women with PCOS, obese women with PCOS have twice the rate of early first-trimester miscarriage. Maternal obesity also increases the risk of congenital anomalies such as neural tube defects, cardiovascular anomalies, and cleft lip and palate. Maternal obesity and fetal macrosomia is associated with increased intrapartum risk, with higher rates of surgical deliveries and complications.

Making the diagnosis of polycystic ovarian syndrome

The first reported description of PCOS was in 1935 by Stein and Leventhal in their report "Amenorrhea associated with bilateral polycystic ovaries." Since that time, there have been many revisions of the diagnostic criteria for PCOS. The most recent consensus for the definition and diagnostic criteria was published in the complete task force report from the International Androgen Excess and PCOS Society in 2009. This most current definition makes hyperandrogenism a key diagnostic feature of PCOS. The most current diagnostic criteria include the following:

1. Hyperandrogenism and/or hirsutism

and

2. Oligo- or anovulation and/or polycystic ovaries

and

3. The exclusion of other androgen excess or androgen-related disorders.

Oligo- or anovulation can most often be diagnosed by menstrual history alone. Some women with PCOS will give a history of "regular" menstrual cycles but are actually experiencing chronic anovulation. In these circumstances, confirmation of ovulation is important is the diagnostic work-up. Ovulation can be confirmed in many ways. Basal body temperature charting or ovulation predictor kits can be used by the patient. These techniques can be difficult to interpret for women with PCOS and are often a source of frustration. An easy method is to obtain a midluteal serum progesterone level between cycle days 21 and 24. A serum progesterone level of over 3 ng/mL confirms ovulation.

The presence of hirsutism, male pattern hair loss, acne, or seborrhea establishes the criteria of clinical hyperandrogenism. Virilization (severe male pattern baldness or hirsutism, clitoromegaly, masculinization of the body habitus) is not typically associated with PCOS, and other etiologies, such as an androgen-secreting tumor or exogenous steroid use, need to be considered. Determination of biochemical hyperandrogenism can be made by obtaining a total testosterone level or a free androgen index and a DHEAS level. Be sure to order a DHEAS and not a dehydroepiandrosterone (DHEA) level, which can sometimes be a source of confusion.

Ovarian size and volume, stromal volume, and antral follicular number are all measures used to describe polycystic ovaries. More than 80% of women with PCOS have either enlarged ovaries on transvaginal ultrasound examination or increased basal antral follicle counts. The presence of polycystic ovaries can be made on sonographic examination by measuring ovarian volume.

☆ TIPS & TRICKS

The determination of antral follicular counts on ultrasound is made in a very specific way. A cursory look at the ovaries with ultrasound and visualizing the classic "string of pearls" was not considered sufficient by the Rotterdam Consensus criteria in 2003. A basal antral follicle (BAF) count consists of a transvaginal ultrasound in the early follicular phase (cycle days 3–5) in a regularly menstruating woman. Irregularly cycling women should have the transvaginal ultrasound performed on cycle days 3–5 following a progestin withdrawal bleed. Antral follicle number should be estimated in both the anteroposterior and the longitudinal cross-sections of the ovaries. The size of follicles smaller than 10 mm should be expressed as the mean of the diameters measured on the two sections (Figure 5.5). If a persistent follicular or corpus luteum cyst is present, the examination for BAF count should wait until the next menstrual cycle. In addition, a BAF count cannot be assessed while a woman is on oral contraceptive pills as these alter the morphology and volume of the ovaries and may lead to inaccurate counts.

Most of the diagnosis of PCOS is determined by clinical examination. The laboratory testing is used to exclude any related androgen disorder or disorder that can cause menstrual irregularities (Table 5.1). Related androgen disorders, such as congenital adrenal hyperplasia, androgen-secreting tumors, severe hyperinsulinemia, and idiopathic hirsutism, are the cause of approximately 10–30% of cases of androgen excess. The measurement of serum total testosterone and DHEAS can rule out ovarian and adrenal tumors. A total testosterone above 150 ng/dL (5.2 nmol/L) or a DHEAS above 700 µg/dL (13.6 µmol/L) may raise the suspicion for ovarian or adrenal androgen-secreting tumors.

Women with nonclassic 21-hydroylase-deficient adrenal hyperplasia can have a similar phenotype to women with severe PCOS. Measurement of serum 17-hydroxyprogesterone (17-OHP), the normal substrate for 21-hydroxylase, is the first screening test for nonclassic 21-hydroxylase deficiency. A morning level greater than 200 ng/dL (6 nmol/L) in the early follicular phase strongly suggests the diagnosis, which may be confirmed by a high-dose (250 µg) adrenocorticotropic hormone stimulation test. Genotyping is now

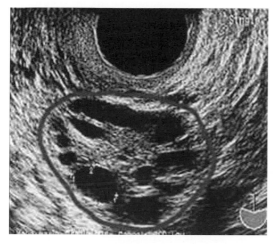

Figure 5.5 Transvaginal ultrasound of a high basal antral follicle count in a woman with polycystic ovarian syndrome.

available to help determine the heterozygosity of the gene in those women who fall in the borderline range in the adrenocorticotropic hormone stimulation test.

Routine screening for Cushing syndrome is not recommended due to the very low prevalence of Cushing syndrome in hyperandrogenic women. Screening for Cushing syndrome should be considered, however, if there is a high clinical suspicion. If a woman presents with rapid weight gain, moon facies, purple striae, thin or easily bruised skin, myopathy, hypertension, or impaired glucose tolerance, the evaluation of androgen excess should include screening for Cushing syndrome with a 24-hour free urinary cortisol measurement.

Common endocrine disorders that may result in menstrual irregularities include hyperprolactinemia and thyroid dysfunction. Elevated prolactin levels are found in approximately 30% of women with secondary amenorrhea. The prevalence of hyperprolactinemia in women with hyperandrogenism, however, is reported to be less than 1% in numerous studies. Similarly, hypothyroidism appears to be much less prevalent in women with hyperandrogenism than previously thought, with a recent prevalence of 0.3%. Despite the low prevalence of thyroid disorders and hyperprolactinemia in women with hyperandrogenism, it is still considered reasonable to screen for these disorders because of the low cost of screening and ease of treatment.

Insulin levels are difficult to measure in clinical settings. Most studies require a euglycemic clamp or frequent intravenous sampling to measure insulin levels, and these methods obviously will not work in an office setting. Largely for that reason, there are currently no recommendations or diagnostic guidelines that address insulin

Table 5.1 Recommended evaluation for polycystic ovarian syndrome

Thyroid-stimulating hormone
Prolactin
Free androgen index or total testosterone
Dehydroepiandrosterone
17-Hydroxyprogesterone
Transvaginal ultrasound with basal antral follicle count

Table 5.2 Criteria for metabolic syndrome (three of five criteria are required)

Abdominal obesity (waist circumference) >88 cm (35 inches)
Triglycerides >150 mg/dL
High-density lipoprotein cholesterol <50 mg/dL
Blood pressure 130/85 mmHg
Fasting and 2-hour glucose from an oral glucose tolerance test 110–126 mg/dL and/or 2-hour glucose 140–199 mg/dL

screening. Some studies suggest that a fasting insulin level of over 80 mU/mL in the fasting state, and/or over 300 mU/mL following a 2- or 3-hour oral glucose tolerance test is diagnostic of insulin resistance. A hemoglobin A_{1c} level above 6.5% is now considered diagnostic of diabetes, but borderline elevations may indicate insulin resistance. Because women with PCOS are at risk for metabolic disorders such as hyperlipidemias, glucose intolerance, and diabetes, the recommendation by the Rotterdam Consensus 2003 is to screen women with PCOS for metabolic syndrome rather than using insulin screening (Table 5.2).

Evaluation of abnormal bleeding in hyperandrogenic women

The evaluation of amenorrhea and oligomenorrhea should include the work-up described above to confirm the underlying diagnosis of PCOS or other related endocrinopathy. A pregnancy test should always be ordered as well. Gonadotropin levels (follicle-stimulating hormone [FSH] and LH) will exclude ovarian failure (a state of high gonadotropin levels) or hypothalamic amenorrhea (a state of low gonadotropin levels); these are often obtained on women with amenorrhea or oligomenorrhea and are sometimes helpful when trying to differentiate a thin woman with PCOS from a hypogonadotropic patient.

If a patient has had a long period of anovulation, an endometrial biopsy should be performed to exclude endometrial hyperplasia and carcinoma. It is of course important to perform a work-up that excludes other potential sources of bleeding. An evaluation of the vulva, vagina, cervix, and uterus should be performed to identify any potential anatomic abnormality such as a vaginal fissure, trauma, foreign bodies, polyp, fibroids, or cancer. Women with PCOS are at risk

of endometrial hyperplasia, so consideration of an endometrial biopsy is indicated even in young women. If an adolescent presents with acute vaginal bleeding at menarche, a work-up for bleeding disorders (e.g., von Willebrand disease, factor deficiencies, platelet dysfunction) should be conducted. One review reported the prevalence of von Willebrand disease in adult women with menorrhagia to be between 5% and 24%, although it is typically not the sole etiology of the menorrhagia. Often an underlying anatomic cause such as a fibroid may contribute to menorrhagia in a woman with a coagulopathy. Less commonly, liver disease can affect sex steroid production and coagulation factors, which may lead to anovulatory bleeding in the setting of a bleeding diathesis.

✋ CAUTION

Consider an endometrial biopsy in a hyperandrogenic, anovulatory woman less than 35 years of age with long periods of amenorrhea or dysfunctional uterine bleeding. Despite her young age, she may be at risk for endometrial hyperplasia or carcinoma. A transvaginal ultrasound is not an adequate tool to assess risk as endometrial stripe measurements have been mostly assessed for postmenopausal risk and not premenopausal risk.

Management of amenorrhea and oligomenorrhea in hyperandrogenic women

Many options are available to treat the chronic oligomenorrhea and amenorrhea experienced by hyperandrogenic women. The main goal is to provide a progestin, in either cyclic or continuous fashion, to prevent endometrial hyperplasia and lower the risk for endometrial carcinoma. One common method is to prescribe a cyclic progestin (such as medroxyprogesterone acetate 10 mg or norethindrone acetate 10 mg for 14 days) to induce regular withdrawal bleeding. The levonorgestrel-releasing intrauterine device may not be sufficient to prevent endometrial growth in women with dysfunctional uterine bleeding diagnosed with endometrial hyperplasia endometrial cancer who wish to preserve fertility.

> ✋ CAUTION
>
> Caution needs to be exercised in this population as there have been a few case reports documenting the development of endometrial carcinoma in the setting of a levonorgestrel-releasing intrauterine device. This dose of progestin may simply not be adequate to fully suppress endometrium in high-risk patients.

The intramuscular or subcutaneous forms of medroxyprogesterone acetate are another choice for women with PCOS. These induce long-term amenorrhea and can effectively treat dysfunctional uterine bleeding and protect the endometrium from the development of hyperplasia and carcinoma.

> ✋ CAUTION
>
> Be careful when prescribing this form of progestin in women with PCOS as there is a high report incidence of weight gain and acne. The median time to ovulation is 10 months from the last injection, which may delay conception for these women. Women with a history of treatment for clinical depression may require closer management on this progestin. Lastly, both of these forms now contain a black box warning from the U.S. Food and Drug Administration to limit use of these forms of progestin to short term only due to the potential irreversible bone mineral density loss.

The subdermal contraceptive etonogestrel implant is another progestin-only long-term treatment for irregular bleeding. The *Physician's Desk Reference* lists precaution when treating hyperlipidemic or glucose-intolerant patients. A review of published studies, however, does not yield any reported adverse impact of the etonogestrel implant on carbohydrate metabolism or lipid profiles. Ovulation occurs approximately 3–4 weeks following removal so it does not delay conception.

Low-dose combination birth control pills containing both estrogen and progestin provide some additional benefits. Low-dose combination pills (<50 μg of ethinylestradiol) not only offer endometrial protection and predictable menses (when given in cyclic fashion), but also provide the benefit of improving the symptoms of hyperandrogenism. The estrogen component increases circulating levels of SHBG, which binds free testosterone and over time will improve acne and hirsutism. The estrogen component also helps ameliorate some of the potential adverse effects of progestins on lipoprotein profiles. The low-dose oral contraceptive pills (OCPs) do not adversely affect carbohydrate metabolism and therefore are not contraindicated in women with hyperinsulinemia. Common side effects of OCPs are nausea, headache, breast tenderness, breakthrough bleeding, and depression.

> ✋ CAUTION
>
> Oral contraceptives should be used with caution in women with hypertension. The main adverse effects are the risk of thrombosis, and smokers and women aged over 35 years are at the greatest risk of thrombosis with their use.

The contraceptive ethinylestradiol/etonogestrel vaginal ring is another option that is usually well received by patients and effective in treating PCOS-related irregular bleeding. The estradiol/etonogestrel vaginal ring appears to have an even lower impact on carbohydrate metabolism than low-dose OCPs. The norelgestromin/ethinylestradiol transdermal contraceptive patch provides similar cycle control and treatment of hyperandrogenism.

✋ CAUTION

Transdermal contraception carries the Food and Drug Administration warning regarding an increased risk of thrombosis compared to oral contraceptive pills. It may also be less effective in women weighing more than 198 lb (90 kg) and therefore should be used cautiously in overweight women with polycystic ovarian syndrome.

Management of severe acute bleeding

Hyperandrogenic women may present with profuse uterine bleeding. Acute bleeding can occur when the uterine lining becomes atrophic, and develops in the setting of metrorrhagia when a woman has continuous, frequent sloughing of the endometrium. In this case, the first-line treatment is estrogen. Estrogen is thought to induce vasoconstriction of the endometrial vessels and aid in platelet aggregation and clotting. It also helps to stimulate growth of the denuded endometrium.

★ TIPS & TRICKS

A tapered regimen of combination oral contraceptives is commonly used and is usually an effective way to arrest bleeding. Four pills are prescribed for 3–4 days, then two pills for 2–3 days, followed by one pill daily to complete a 21-day course. The use of an oral contraceptive taper in this setting may exacerbate bleeding due to the progestin effect. A recommended protocol is to prescribe oral conjugated equine estrogen 2.5 mg every 6 hours. Bleeding is usually controlled within 24 hours. If it is not, a higher dose (5 mg) every 6 hours can be prescribed, or intravenous estrogen can be administered. Intravenous conjugated equine estrogen is administered at a dose of 25 mg every 4 hours, and a response usually occurs within three doses. There are no studies showing any

advantage of intravenous administration over oral administration. All of these regimens may elicit nausea and vomiting due to the high dose of estrogen. An antiemetic should be prescribed along with the estrogen therapy. It is critical that any estrogen therapy be followed with a progestin for 14 days to bring about a withdrawal bleed.

A dilatation and curettage (D&C) may be performed if hormonal therapy is not effective or if a woman is hemodynamically unstable and requires immediate treatment. A D&C also provides a pathologic diagnosis to rule out endometrial hyperplasia or carcinoma. It is, however, a temporary treatment for severe menorrhagia: it will not correct the chronic problem, and the woman will still benefit from long-term hormonal therapy. Other surgical options include endometrial ablation, uterine artery embolization, and hysterectomy. Obviously, these three surgical options should be avoided in women of reproductive age desirous of future childbearing.

Management of metabolic dysfunction

Lifestyle interventions

The most effective treatment of the endocrine and metabolic disorders associated with PCOS is through behavior modification, including diet and exercise. It is important to convey to patients that behavioral modification alone is more effective than pharmacologic treatments.

⚛ SCIENCE REVISITED

The Diabetes Prevention Program Research Group reported that lifestyle intervention alone was significantly more effective at reducing risk of diabetes than administration of metformin. The lifestyle intervention reduced the incidence of diabetes by 58% and metformin reduced it by 31% compared to controls. This study did not specifically use subjects with polycystic ovarian syndrome (PCOS), but their subjects had similar risk factors for development of diabetes, namely being overweight or obese subjects with impaired glucose intolerance. A 10-year follow-up of this population showed that the although both metformin and lifestyle intervention were associated with a long-term reduction in the development of type 2 diabetes, the group that instituted lifestyle changes showed the great cumulative benefit. Weight loss through diet and exercise will be a lifelong struggle for many women with PCOS. Based on these and similar data, it is important for healthcare providers to continue to encourage overweight and obese women with PCOS to maintain lifestyle modification for the most effective long-term treatment of the metabolic and endocrinologic sequelae.

Only about half of overweight patients are told by their primary care physician that their health problems are associated with being overweight, and about half of these receive counseling about diet and exercise. It can be difficult for the busy health provider to take time to counsel. Often there is an assumption that another primary care provider has already counseled the patient or that the patient may view the counseling as nagging, or the provider may not feel adequately educated in weight counseling. One strategy is to develop a connection to a reputable weight loss center that can provide nutritional and exercise counseling. Often weight loss centers can address some of the other support required by overweight and obese women, such as support groups or psychologists.

When discussing the effect of weight on PCOS, it is often encouraging for a woman to hear that very little weight loss can yield considerable benefits. For instance, the Diabetes Prevention Program designed the diet and exercise program for at least 7% body weight loss. One widely cited Australian study, however, showed that as little as a 2–5% reduction in body weight over 6 months yielded a 70% improvement in insulin sensitivity, and this was associated with the return of reproductive function, with a 50% resumption of ovulation in previously anovulatory women and an 11% spontaneous pregnancy rate. A 12-week moderate caloric restriction to 1200 kcal daily and moderate exercise three times weekly showed

an almost 80% improvement in menses, with almost 10% becoming eumenorrheic. An overweight or obese woman may feel that the aim of weight loss is too daunting when, in fact, it should be approached as a series of small attainable goals.

Lifestyle modification with weight loss not only reduces hyperinsulinemia, decreases androgen levels, and corrects reproductive parameters such as menstrual cyclicity, ovulation and fecundity, but also helps ameliorate many of the other medical consequences of PCOS. Sleep apnea and dyslipidemias are improved with weight loss. Increased preconception physical activity reduces the development of glucose intolerance and gestational diabetes. Quality of life measures such as self-esteem and sense of wellbeing are improved as well. Given all these benefits, it is important to remain an advocate for your patient through continued encouragement during periods of plateauing or weight gain, and through praise during times of successful weight loss.

A comprehensive, multidisciplinary approach to weight loss can help facilitate and encourage long-term success. Lifestyle modifications require changes in both diet and exercise. Pharmacologic and psychological support is often an important adjunct to behavioral changes. Consultation with a nutritionist and/or personal trainer can help motivate and guide a patient to successful weight loss. Lastly, bariatric procedures are indicated in some circumstances.

Diet

Often the question is posed of what diet is best for women with PCOS. The current literature is abundant with studies comparing specific diet types for the treatment of obesity, with conflicting results. Early Cochrane Reviews supported low-glycemic diets compared to calorie-restricted diets for promotion of weight loss and improvement of metabolic parameters. A more recent Cochrane Review demonstrated no advantage between fat-restricted and calorie-restricted diets, and a recent large 2-year trial in the *New England Journal of Medicine* revealed no clinical significance in weight loss regardless of which macronutrients were emphasized in the diet.

Relatively few studies have examined the optimal diet for women with PCOS. Reduced carbohydrate intake improved fasting insulin levels and acute insulin response to glucose in women with PCOS. Other studies have demonstrated a short-term reduction in androgen levels in women with PCOS following a low-fat, high-fiber meal or a high-protein diet compared to a typical high-fat meal. Most of the studies looking at the effect of specific diets on androgen levels in women with PCOS are short in duration. When reviewing all the data regarding long-term weight loss effects, it seems clear that the specific diet is not terribly important. Therefore, an overweight or obese woman with PCOS should be counseled to find healthy dietary modifications that she can maintain. The low-carbohydrate diet may be a little more effective in the short term (3–6 months), but all diets appear equivalent over the long term (1 year or more). The diet the woman likes best and can adhere to is the one that is best for her.

Exercise

It is important to provide women with specific recommendations for exercise rather than saying simply to become more active. Since 1995, when the Centers for Disease Control published exercise guidelines, the common advice has been that adults obtain at least 30 minutes of moderate-intensity physical activity on 5 or more days a week, for a total of at least 150 minutes a week.

> ### ⬡ SCIENCE REVISITED
>
> In 2008, the National Institutes of Health Department of Health and Human Services issued new guidelines for physical activity for Americans. Current guidelines for all Americans show no significant difference between 30 minutes of exercise on 5 or more days or 150 minutes of exercise divided into either fewer or more days. The total time is what is considered important. New recommendations suggest that all people exercise at least 150 minutes (2 hours and 30 minutes) a week at moderate intensity, or 75 minutes (1 hour and 15 minutes) a week of vigorous intensity aerobic physical activity, or an equivalent combination of both moderate and vigorous aerobic activity.

People who want to lose more than 5% of their body weight and people who are trying to maintain a weight loss require more physical activity unless they also reduce their caloric intake. Recommendation by the National Institutes of Health Department of Health and Human Services for these people is to do more than 300 minutes of moderate intensity activity a week to meet weight control goals.

> ### ⬛ TIPS & TRICKS
>
> The easiest way to counsel patients about intensity of exercise is to discuss the concept of relative intensity, that is, have a person pay attention to their level of exertion. In general, a person doing moderate-intensity aerobic activity can talk, but not sing. A person doing vigorous intensity activity cannot say more than a few words without getting short of breath. Examples of moderate-intensity exercise include brisk walking, ballroom dancing, gardening, and water aerobics. Examples of vigorous intensity include jogging, running, jumping ropes, and swimming laps.

There are few studies looking at exercise alone for treatment of PCOS, but most lifestyle intervention studies include both diet and exercise. A study using a rodent model of PCOS did show improved ovarian morphology and decreased serum androgen levels in rats that increased their exercise level without modifying their diet. One study of women with PCOS demonstrated improved lipoprotein particle composition with institution of moderate-intensity exercise alone. Another study examining continuous versus intermittent aerobic exercise in patients with metabolic syndrome reported similar benefits of weight loss, improved insulin sensitivity, and decreased blood pressure. Exercise has been shown to reduce risk for diabetes in many populations at high risk by reducing insulin resistance. These studies usually include men and women with metabolic syndrome, who are at similar risks to women with PCOS.

Exercise improves insulin sensitivity by increasing the uptake of glucose at the muscular level, resulting in a compensatory decline in insulin secretion. Vigorous aerobic-intensity exercise has been shown to have the most significant effect on insulin sensitivity. Weight resistance two to three times per week has also been shown to improve markers associated with insulin sensitivity such as C-reactive protein and adiponectin and improvement in glycated hemoglobin in diabetics. Given these data, is seems reasonable to encourage overweight and obese women with PCOS to engage in at least 300 minutes of aerobic exercise weekly, with additional time devoted to weight resistance two to three times weekly. Prescribed weight loss guidelines yield more weight loss and improvements in psychological outcomes compared to general lifestyle advice in young overweight or obese women. Therefore it is important to quantify exercise and diet advice rather than speak in generalities to these patients.

Recommendations for women of normal BMI with PCOS are a little less clear. Exercise clearly has benefits on insulin sensitivity in nonobese women. In a normal-weight woman with PCOS, the goal of exercise is to enhance her metabolic and endocrine profile without necessarily inducing weight loss. Therefore, the Department of Health and Human Services recommendation for general physical activity for 150 minutes each week seems appropriate.

Psychological support

Despite many medical studies reporting the adverse impact of PCOS on the women's emotional and mental health, there are very few studies addressing appropriate interventions. A nurse-led peer support group helps reduce social isolation, provide information, and instill a feeling of empowerment to women with PCOS. A clinician should address and ask about clinical depression and anxiety and be prepared to treat accordingly, with pharmacologic interventions when appropriate. Partnering the patient with a psychologist or therapist can help to treat and modify many of the mood disorders that affect the quality of life of these women. An experienced therapist may be very instrumental in helping identify patterns and triggers of binge eating or emotional eating that may be exacerbating the symptoms of PCOS. Acupuncture has been widely studied and is effective in decreasing anxiety scores in women undergoing fertility treatment. Although these studies did not specifically address PCOS, it can be extrapolated that this technique would likely help to alleviate stress scores in women with PCOS as well.

Insulin-sensitizing agents

The most widely studied insulin-sensitizing agents used to treat PCOS are metformin and the glitazones. Insulin-sensitizing agents have been shown to improve many of the metabolic and endocrine disorders associated with PCOS.

Administration of metformin

Metformin is a biguanide oral antihyperglycemic agent. It works by decreasing hepatic glucose production and intestinal absorption of glucose. It also improves insulin sensitivity by increasing peripheral glucose uptake and utilization. It does not induce hypoglycemia and may be used in patients who self-describe having symptoms they associate with low blood sugar.

> **⚠ CAUTION**
>
> Metformin can cause many side effects, mostly related to gastrointestinal distress. Common side effects include diarrhea, flatulence, indigestion, nausea, vomiting, and loose stools. The rare adverse effect associated with metformin is lactic acidosis, which carries a 50% mortality risk. The cases of lactic acidosis reported with metformin use were not in otherwise healthy women with polycystic ovarian syndrome. These cases were reported in patients with complicated medical histories such as diabetes, heart failure, or significant renal or hepatic disease. A patient should be counseled to avoid excessive alcohol consumption as alcohol potentiates the effect of metformin on lactic acidosis. It is common practice to check a complete chemistry panel in women prior to initiating metformin. Serum creatinine level over 1.4 mg/dL is considered a contraindication for women taking metformin, and precaution is advised if a woman has elevated liver enzymes.

Metformin should be held for 48 hours following HSG, any radiologic examination that requires use of intravenous contrast media. There are no clear guidelines for its use during a hystero/salpingogram (HSG). Contrast media is injected into the uterine cavity during an HSG and not directly administered intravenously, but it may intravasate into uterine vessels during the procedure. For this reason, have the patient hold her dose of metformin the day prior to the HSG.

The dosage of metformin used in most published studies is a maximal dose of 1,500–2,000 mg a day administered orally in divided doses. The gastrointestinal side effects of metformin can be mitigated by prescribing a tapering dose. It is best tolerated if taken with food. Prescribe 500 mg for 1 week to be taken at breakfast. If this is tolerated, the patient increases the dose to 500 mg at breakfast and dinner. She can then increase the dose each week by 500 mg at mealtimes until the maximum dose of 2,000 mg is achieved. If she finds a maximum dose intolerable, simply have her reduce the dose by 500 mg to one she can tolerate. Gastrointestinal symptoms are often exacerbated by the ingestion of fatty and high carbohydrate foods, so proper counseling of metformin usage can also help with adherence to a healthy diet.

Effect of metformin metabolic and endocrine parameters in women with polycystic ovarian syndrome

Numerous studies have reported a reduction in hyperinsulinemia, LH levels, and free testosterone concentrations with metformin treatment in overweight women with polycystic ovaries. Metformin clearly improves ovulatory rates and menstrual disturbances in obese women with PCOS. A Cochrane Review in 2009 showed almost twice the ovulatory rate in women with PCOS taking metformin as occurred in controls. OCPs, however, are more effective than metformin at improving menstrual patterns. Data suggest that even women with PCOS who are of normal body weight benefit from metformin administration.

Hirsutism, biochemical hyperandrogenism, and insulin sensitivity improve in lean women with PCOS taking metformin, as do ovulatory and menstrual patterns.

Effect of metformin on fertility and pregnancy

Metformin is a Food and Drug Administration (FDA) Pregnancy Category B drug, while the glitazones are Pregnancy Category C drugs. For this reason, most physicians are comfortable prescribing metformin to women with PCOS who are trying to conceive. The other insulin-sensitizing agents are good options in women with PCOS who are not trying to conceive. The Pregnancy in Polycystic Ovary Syndrome trial (PPCOS) in 2007 was the definitive multicenter trial looking at live birth rates of women with PCOS taking metformin alone, clomiphene citrate alone, or a combination of both drugs.

⋆ TIPS & TRICKS

The Pregnancy in Polycystic Ovary Syndrome trial and a Cochrane Review from 2009 conclude that metformin alone does not appear to improve live birth rates compared to clomiphene citrate. Metformin does appear, however, to reduce the incidence of ovarian hyperstimulation in in-vitro fertilization cycles.

Metformin has been shown in some early studies to significantly reduce the incidence of miscarriage in women with PCOS and improve the risk of developing gestational diabetes. A recent systematic review of the literature, however, demonstrated no significant impact of metformin on risk of abortion in women with PCOS. It may, therefore, be prudent to continue metformin to help reduce the risk of gestational diabetes. It is now common practice to continue women with PCOS on metformin through the first trimester, and some obstetricians may elect to continue it throughout pregnancy. Metformin has been used for decades in South Africa throughout pregnancy without any reported teratogenicity or adverse neonatal effects. Metformin is currently not approved by the FDA for use in pregnancy, and large multicenter trials need to investigate the effect on rates of miscarriage and gestational diabetes.

Other insulin-sensitizing agents

The glitazones (troglitazone, rosiglitazone, pioglitazone) and D-chiro-inositol (DCI) have been studied in the treatment of PCOS. The glitazones bind and activate the nuclear receptor peroxisome proliferator-activated receptor gamma (PPAR-gamma). PPAR-gamma plays an important function in regulating energy homeostasis and increases insulin sensitivity at the level of muscle and adipose tissue.

Troglitazone is effective for reducing insulin levels and hyperandrogenisim but was taken off the worldwide market in 2000 due to cases of hepatic necrosis. Pioglitazone and rosiglitazone remain available and are a good alternative to metformin in women with PCOS who are not pregnant, especially women who are unable to tolerate the gastrointestinal side effects of metformin. The glitazones tend to have better tolerance than metformin. Dosing of pioglitazone is commonly 30–45 mg once daily in women with PCOS. The dose of rosiglitazone is 4 mg twice daily.

> ### ⚠ CAUTION
>
> The glitazones can exacerbate edema and need to be used cautiously in patients with heart failure. A dose-related small weight gain has been seen with both of these drugs. Some data suggests a risk of bone fractures with use of long-term rosiglitazone.

Unlike metformin, which does not exacerbate hypoglycemia, the glitazones may cause hypoglycemic periods. Liver function tests should be checked prior to the initiation of either agent. Both pioglitazone and rosiglitazone improve insulin sensitivity, improve hyperandrogenism, and increase SHBG concentrations in both lean and obese women with PCOS. There are small studies that show improved spontaneous pregnancy rates. The glitazones have also been shown to improve ovulatory rates in women with PCOS who were previously clomiphene resistant, but there has not been a large multicenter trial like the PPCOS trial evaluating the effect on live birth rate. Combined rosiglitazone and metformin has not yielded any significant additive effect in treatment outcomes. Rosiglitazone has shown slightly improved effects on androgen levels, clinical hirsutism, and menstrual disturbances compared to metformin.

The antidiabetic drug exenatide is an analog of the hormone incretin (glucagon-like peptide 1). It increases insulin secretion, increases beta-cell growth, slows gastric emptying, and may decrease food intake. One report of exenatide demonstrated improved menstrual cyclicity and endocrine and metabolic parameters with combined metformin and exenatide administration in women with PCOS compared to either agent alone. Exenatide is commonly prescribed as 5 μg subcutaneously twice daily for 4 weeks and then increased to 10 μg subcutaneously twice daily. Common adverse effects include hypoglycemia and gastrointestinal disturbances.

Inositolphosphoglycan mediators play a role in insulin secretion. There is evidence that one of the mechanism of insulin resistance in women with PCOS is related to altered inositolphosphoglycan function, which in turn leads to decreased DCI levels and insulin resistance. Oral supplementation with 1,200 mg DCI showed improved measurements of insulin sensitivity, improved serum androgen levels, decreased blood pressure, and improved lipid profiles in both obese and lean women with PCOS. This drug, however, has not been evaluated by the FDA for safety in pregnancy.

Chromium improves insulin sensitivity through its action on kinase activity of the insulin receptor. Chromium picolinate, administered orally as 200 μg daily for 4 months improved glucose tolerance but did not appear to have an effect on menstrual or hormonal parameters of women with PCOS.

Cinnamon extract improves insulin sensitivity by enhancing insulin signaling via phosphoinositol 3-kinase activity. Oral cinnamon extract was shown to reduce fasting glucose and improve lipid profiles in diabetic subjects. In women with PCOS, a pilot study showed improved fasting and

2-hour oral glucose tolerance tests. BMI, testosterone, and estradiol levels, however, remained unchanged. Its effect on ovulatory and menstrual pattern has not been well studied.

Weight loss agents in polycystic ovarian syndrome

Several weight loss agents have been used in women with PCOS. Orlistat binds to gastric and pancreatic lipases, blocking the absorption of triglycerides. This results in sustained weight loss with improved glycemic and lipid profiles. Women with PCOS administered orlistat orally 120 mg three times daily had significant weight loss, improved total testosterone and free androgen index, and insulin sensitivity improved only with short-term treatment; extended treatment did not show a significant change in androgen levels or insulin resistance. Effects on hormonal and menstrual parameters were not studied.

⚠ CAUTION

Orlistat has significant gastrointestinal side effects including steatorrhea and fecal incontinence, and therefore is often poorly tolerated by patients.

Improved insulin sensitivity in women with PCOS on sibutramine appears to be directly related to the degree of weight loss. Improved serum androgen level and clinical hirsutism were noted with sibutramine 15 mg orally once daily. Endocrine and menstrual parameters have not been measured. Sibutramine acts via adrenergic, serotonergic, and dopaminergic pathways to induce weight loss.

⚠ CAUTION

Sibutramine cannot be used in patients with severe renal or hepatic dysfunction, and there is a long list of adverse interactions with other drugs. Close monitoring of pulse and blood pressure is advised when prescribing this drug. It is a Food and Drug Administration Pregnancy Category C drug and should not be used in pregnant women.

Surgical management of polycystic ovarian syndrome

Surgical interventions are at times indicated for treating women with PCOS. Bariatric surgery may be recommended in women with PCOS who have a BMI equal or greater than 40kg/m^2 or if they have a BMI between 35 and 40 and suffer a medical condition that is exacerbated by their weight. Ovarian drilling is another surgical option indicated for treating PCOS and can be considered an adjunct or alternative to medical therapy. Ovarian drilling is indicated in treating PCOS regardless of weight.

Bariatric surgery for polycystic ovarian syndrome

There are two general types of bariatric procedure for the treatment of obesity: restrictive and malabsorptive procedures. Restrictive procedures are performed to restrict a portion of the stomach, thereby reducing the size of the stomach and limiting the amount of food a person can eat at one time. The most common restrictive procedure performed now is laparoscopic gastric banding, which compartmentalizes the upper stomach by placing a tight, adjustable silicon ring around the entrance to the stomach. The laparoscopic banding procedure reduces body weight by about 45–70% of excess weight over 2 years. The other restrictive procedure is the sleeve gastrectomy, which is usually reserved for patients with extreme obesity whose BMI is equal to or greater than 50kg/m^2. The sleeve gastrectomy involves removal of most of the stomach, leaving a narrow area of the stomach. This procedure is often performed as the first step in bariatric procedures to allow for initial weight loss. The patient can then undergo a malabsorptive surgery at a later time. The sleeve gastrectomy typically results in a 30% loss of excess weight over 2 years.

Malabsorptive procedures decrease the length of small intestine, thereby limiting the amount of nutrients and calories absorbed by the body. The jejunoileal bypass and the biliopancreatic diversion are both types of the malabsorptive procedures. The roux-en-Y gastric bypass (RYBG) has both restrictive and malabsorptive effects and remains one of the most commonly performed bariatric procedures. It is classically performed with an abdominal incision but has been conducted laparoscopically as well. The RYGB is performed by dividing the stomach and attaching a small stomach pouch directly to the small intestine, bypassing part of the duodenum. Weight loss in the first year following RYGB is approximately 65% of excess weight.

Anovulatory bleeding and oligomenorrhea is very common in obese women prior to bariatric surgery. Almost 70% of women who undergo bariatric surgery experience a restoration of menstrual cyclicity. Women who have greater weight loss following the surgery are more likely to become ovulatory. Bariatric surgery also improves metabolic syndrome in obese patients regardless of the type of procedure performed. Both the restrictive and the malabsorptive surgeries lead to improved anthropomorphic measures (waist-to-hip ratio, BMI), fasting glucose, triglyceride levels, and lipid profile. About 80% of patients will have complete resolution of diabetes and improved hypertension, and about 85% of patients undergoing bariatric surgery will have resolution or improvement of sleep apnea.

ventral hernias. Patients undergoing bariatric surgery are followed up closely afterward by nutritionists and clinicians to guard for nutritional and metabolic disorders. Dumping syndrome and hypoglycemia can also occur. Postbariatric patients will require lifelong supplementation with multivitamins and supplements such as vitamin B_{12}, thiamine, and folate. Studies of pregnancies following the malabsorptive procedures of jejunoileal bypass and biliopancreatic diversion have reported increased rates of low birth weight, preterm deliveries, and intrauterine growth restriction. The laparoscopic adjustable band has lower perinatal morbidity. Generally, the recommendation is for a woman to wait 1–2 years following bariatric procedures before trying to conceive.

Ovarian drilling for polycystic ovarian syndrome

Surgical management of PCOS dates back to the 1930s, when bilateral ovarian wedge resections were performed as a means of reducing the stromal mass of the ovaries and restoring ovulation. Laparoscopic ovarian surgery has now replaced the open wedge resection. Several laparoscopic methods have been described for the treatment of PCOS. The most common procedure is laparoscopic ovarian drilling, which can be performed with either laser or electrocautery. Use of electrocautery is the more widespread procedure. A unipolar laparoscopic needle is introduced about 1–2 cm into the ovarian stroma (Figure 5.6). Between approximately four and six needle punctures are applied to each ovary to induce thermal damage to the underlying stroma, which is responsible for androgen production.

Laparoscopic ovarian drilling restores ovulation in about 50% of women and is associated with a significant improvement in menstrual regularity. Decreases in androgen levels are reported, and the LH-to-FSH ratio normalizes following the procedure. Reports are mixed regarding the effect of laparoscopic drilling on insulin sensitivity. Ovulatory rates and rates of ongoing pregnancy were inversely tied to the BMI of the patient undergoing the procedure. Laparoscopic ovarian drilling is far less successful in treating

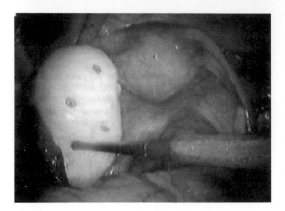

Figure 5.6 Laparoscopic ovarian drilling (see Plate 5.6).

infertility in women who are obese or have other factors contributing to their infertility. It is indicated for clomiphene-resistant women. About half of women who undergo ovarian drilling will conceive in the following year. The pregnancy rates following the drilling procedure are equivalent to gonadotropin administration without putting the patient at the increased risk for multiple births and ovarian hyperstimulation.

> ✋ **CAUTION**
>
> The risks of drilling include the surgery-related risks of anesthesia, bleeding, infection, injury to nearby organs, and postsurgical adhesion formation. Laparoscopic drilling does not appear to adversely affect ovarian reserve.

Treatment of hyperandrogenism

The first-line treatment for women with clinical hyperandrogenism (hirsutism and acne) is usually OCPs, as described above. OCPs improve acne and hirsutism via several mechanisms. The estrogen component of OCPs increases the concentrations of SHBG, thereby lowering free testosterone levels. OCPs also suppress LH, the primary stimulus for ovarian androgen production. Most hyperandrogenic women on OCPs report significant hair reduction. The third-generation progestins levonorgestrel, desogestrel, norgestimate, and gestodene have a more dramatic impact on serum levels of SHBG and testosterone compared to other forms of progestins, but the clinical response to hirsutism appears to be about the same regardless of the form of low-dose OCP administered.

The progestin drospirenone is a derivative of spironolactone and both antiandrogen and antimineralocorticoid activity and is available in the OCPs Yasmin and Yaz. The antiandrogen effect of the drospirenone is not as powerful as spironolactone and has the same clinical effect as other OCPs.

> ☆ **TIPS & TRICKS**
>
> It is important to remind the patient that decreased hair growth may not be clinically apparent for up to 6 months due to the life cycle of the hair follicle. If a woman does not see improvement after a 6-month trial of oral contraceptives, the addition of an antiandrogen medication is suggested.

Cyproterone acetate is a 17-hydroxyprogesterone derivative that blocks dihydrotestosterone and competes for the androgen receptor. It is used as the progestin in the combination OCPs Diane, Diane 35, and Dianette with ethinylestradiol of varying doses. Cyproterone acetate can also be used at higher doses of 12.5–100 mg daily on cycle days 5–14 as monotherapy with sequential ethinylestradiol. The clinical effect of the lower-dose OCP Dianette has similar results to the high-dose sequential method. Common side effects include fatigue, weight gain, and decreased libido. It is contraindicated in patients with liver disease and a history of thrombosis, and should be administered with precaution in patients with a history of renal dysfunction, heart disease, and depression. Cyproterone is widely available worldwide except in the United States.

The antiandrogen medications are highly effective at improving cosmesis but need to be prescribed in conjunction with a birth control agent. There is potential teratogenic risk to a male fetus if a woman conceives while on antiandrogen medication. There may also be a slight additive effect of combining an OCP with an antiandrogen for the treatment of hirsutism. These pharmacologic agents act via different mechanisms, and one study showed a slight improvement with combined therapy.

⚙ SCIENCE REVISITED

Spironolactone, an aldosterone and androgen receptor antagonist, is the most commonly used antiandrogen. It reduces androgen levels by lowering levels of the enzymes 17-hydroxylase and 17,20-lyase, as well as the enzymes involved in the early steps of androgen synthesis. Spironolactone also competitively binds to dihydrotestosterone receptors in peripheral tissues such as the hair follicles.

Spironolactone has been shown to improve hirsutism in about 60–70% of androgenic women. It is dosed in a titrated manner with a usual starting oral dose of 50 mg twice daily and can be increased in 50 mg increments to a maximal dose of 100 mg twice daily. Decreased hirsutism is typically experienced in 2–5 months.

✋ CAUTION

Spironolactone is typically well tolerated but can be associated with several adverse effects. Side effects include headache, increased body weight, polyuria, increased appetite, weakness, and fatigue. Hyperkalemia is a rare occurrence. Postural hypotension resulting from diuresis may also occur. Dose-dependent menstrual irregularities and menorrhagia can also occur with spironolactone. Menstrual irregularities can be best controlled by prescribed dual therapy with oral contraceptive pills. If a woman is unable to take oral contraceptives and is using a different form of contraception while on spironolactone, the drug can be administered on cycle days 4–21 to allow a synchronized withdrawal bleed. Spironolactone is contraindicated in women with renal and liver impairment. It carries a Food and Drug Administration black box warning due to the tumorigenicity seen in rat studies and therefore should be prescribed in the lowest effective daily dose.

Other antiandrogen medications include finasteride, a competitive inhibitor of 5-alpha reductase, and the enzyme that catalyzes the conversion of testosterone to DHT. Due to its high teratogenic potential, it is imperative that a woman is on a form of contraception if this drug is prescribed.

✋ CAUTION

There is potential teratogenicity even if a pregnant woman simply handles finasteride, through its skin absorption, and it should be used with caution. It is most commonly prescribed as doses of 5 mg orally for treatment of hirsutism, although some studies have used a 7.5 mg daily dose. Finasteride is contraindicated in women with liver impairment or an obstructive uropathy. Side effects include gastrointestinal disturbance such as constipation or diarrhea. Thrombocytopenia and skin rashes have been reported.

Flutamide, a nonsteroidal antiandrogen, is an androgen receptor antagonist. The oral dose most commonly used to treat hirsutism is 250 mg daily, but doses as high as 375 mg daily have been used in some studies.

✋ CAUTION

Common side effects of flutamide include skin rashes, sweating, and gastrointestinal symptoms such as diarrhea and nausea. Serious adverse effects include hepatotoxicity, thrombocytopenia, anemia, and leukopenia. Flutamide is contraindicated in patients with hepatic impairment. The risk for hepatotoxicity may be dose related as it has not been reported in the low doses typically administered for treatment of hirsutism. Despite this, serum transaminase levels need to be monitored prior to treatment, every month for the first 4 months, and then periodically thereafter.

Most studies show a similar reduction in hirsutism when comparing spironolactone, flutamide, and finasteride. A few studies have demonstrated improved efficacy with flutamide, but the data are limited. Given the expense of flutamide and finasteride as well as the potential hepatotoxicity of flutamide, the first-line antiandrogen treatment should be spironolactone.

Eflornithine (marketed as Vaniqa) is a topical cream that blocks the enzyme ornithine decarboxylase in skin and acts by inhibiting follicular cell growth and reducing the rate of hair growth. Eflornithine needs to be applied twice daily, with at least 8 hours between each application, to clean, dry skin, and left on for 4 hours. It can be applied under make-up. It produces a temporary inhibition, and hair regrows after cessation of application within about 8 weeks. It is generally well tolerated with few adverse effects. Topical antiandrogen creams such as canrenone and topical finasteride are of very limited benefit and are generally not suggested.

Other medical treatments for hirsutism play a lesser role. The insulin-sensitizing agents metformin and rosiglitazone have been shown to reduce serum levels of androgens, but in a recent meta-analysis they did not uniformly improve clinical hirsutism when Ferrimen–Gallwey scores were evaluated. In fact, the 2008 recommendations by the Endocrine Society Clinical Practice Guideline

advised against the use of insulin-sensitizing agents for the treatment of hirsutism.

Glucocorticoids have been used to treat women with nonclassical congenital adrenal hyperplasia for ovulation induction. The use of glucocorticoids for women with hirsutism due to other causes is not suggested. Gonadotropin-releasing hormone agonists, such as leuprolide acetate, are reserved for severely hyperandrogenic women who have not had an adequate response to oral contraceptives and antiandrogen therapy.

The pharmacologic agents will not improve existing hair but only decrease future hair growth. The best treatments for the reduction of hair that is already present are mechanical hair removal treatments such as shaving, depilatory creams, waxing, threading, electrolysis, and photoepilation (laser and intense pulsed light). Chemical depilatory creams are very commonly used due to their ease and low cost. They can cause a chemical dermatitis but are generally well tolerated. Plucking, threading, and waxing are epilation treatments to remove hair to the level of the follicle bulb and are also safe methods that are inexpensive and can be performed in the privacy of a patient's home, although they involve some discomfort for the patient.

Both laser and electrolysis treatments are marketed as permanent forms of hair removal, but many patients will experience hair regrowth so these therefore should be considered forms of hair reduction. Laser therapy works by destroying hair through photothermolysis, primarily by targeting the melanin in the hair bulb. The efficacy of laser and photoepilation treatment is based on studies largely with poor methodology. A recent Cochrane Review reported a short-term effect of about 50% hair reduction with alexandrite and diode lasers up to 6 months after treatment. Little evidence was obtained for an effect of intense pulsed light or ND:YAG or ruby laser. Typically, women require four to six treatments at about 6-week intervals with photoepilation, and it is costly. After a year, there is generally a return of vellus hair, and "touch-up" treatments may be necessary. Improved results have been seen when eflornithine was administered in conjunction with laser treatment.

Electrolysis is a physical method of hair removal that has been used since 1875 and works by destroying the hair follicle with an electric current. It is a form of permanent hair reduction, and about 25–50% of the hair regrows after 6 months. When comparing laser and electrolysis, laser therapy demonstrated a 70% reduction in hair count, whereas electrolysis demonstrated a 35% reduction over 6 months.

> ### ✋ CAUTION
>
> Both laser and electrolysis procedures can be painful so pretreatment with a topical anesthetic agent may be useful. Rarely, scarring or pigment change can occur with these methods.

Ovulation induction for polycystic ovarian syndrome

The goal of ovulation induction in women with hyperandrogenic ovulatory disorders is to restore ovulation with monofollicular development. Clomiphene citrate is the first-line agent and has been used since the 1950s.

> ### ⚛ SCIENCE REVISITED
>
> Clomiphene is a triphenylethylene derivative that acts as a selective estrogen receptor modulator with both competitive agonist and antagonist activity depending on the target tissue. It primarily acts on the hypothalamus to provide negative feedback by binding to estrogen receptors. A compensatory surge of follicle-stimulating hormone and luteinizing hormone is released from the pituitary, thereby stimulating ovulation.

Clomiphene is very effective in inducing ovulation in women with PCOS. About 70% of anovulatory women will ovulate in response to clomiphene, and about 40% will conceive. The majority of pregnancies occur in the first 6 months of usage. The starting dose of clomiphene is 50 mg taken orally beginning on cycle days 2, 3, 4, or 5 for a 5-day course. Often, a progestin withdrawal bleed is required to first elicit menses.

Ovulation can then be determined by use of basal body temperature charting, ovulation predictor kits, transvaginal ultrasound monitoring, or midluteal progesterone. The dose is increased by 50 mg increments up to a maximal dose of 250 mg daily until the ovulatory dose is achieved. Women with PCOS, especially overweight or obese women, may be less responsive to clomiphene and require higher doses. Once the ovulatory dose has been determined, there is no need to further increase the dosage.

Clomiphene-resistant women may benefit from a prolonged course of clomiphene for up to 8 days, and the addition of a glucocorticoid has been shown to help in hyperandrogenic women. Metformin improves ovulatory rates but does not improve live birth rates. Intercourse or insemination can then be timed to ovulation.

> ### ✋ CAUTION
>
> Common side effects include hot flashes, nausea, mood swings, and irritability. Ovarian enlargement may be experienced as bloating, abdominal discomfort, or pressure. Headaches or vision changes may occur but are rare. Most of the time, visual disturbances such as scotomas are reversible, but there have been reports of persisting symptoms. In some women, the antiestrogenic effect of clomiphene can decrease cervical mucus or interfere with endometrial development. The main risk is multiple gestations: there is about a 10% chance of twins, but higher-order multiples are rare with clomiphene. There is no increased risk of birth defects or miscarriage with the drug.

One common alternative to clomiphene for ovulation induction is the use of the aromatase inhibitors letrozole and anastrazole. The typical starting dose of letrozole is 2.5 mg orally on cycle days 3–7. If ovulation is not achieved with this dose, it can be increased in 2.5 mg increments up to 7.5 mg to achieve ovulation.

Direct comparisons of clomiphene to letrozole did not demonstrate any difference in risk for birth defects when administered carefully. The aromatase inhibitors tend to have fewer side effects than clomiphene, which may improve tolerability. The largest studies evaluating letrozole demonstrated favorable pregnancy rates compared to both clomiphene and gonadotropins, with a significantly decreased rate of multiple gestations.

The goals of gonadotropin therapy for treatment of hyperandrogenic anovulatory disorders are to induce ovulation with monofollicular development rather than superovulation. Gonadotropin therapy may be considered if a woman is not responsive to oral ovulation induction agents. Highly purified human menopausal gonadotropin or recombinant FSH is now used. Human menopausal gonadotropin is administered intramuscularly, and recombinant FSH is administered subcutaneously. Both are prescribed as daily injections beginning on cycle day 3 until a mature follicle is visualized by transvaginal ultrasound monitoring and adequate serum estradiol levels have been achieved.

Pregnancy rates are approximately 20% per cycle and overall 40% per patient. The main risk of gonadotropin therapy is an approximately 25% risk of multiple gestations.

IVF is widely becoming the second-line therapy if a woman with PCOS has failed ovulation induction with the oral agents. IVF has a higher per cycle live birth rate than COH, with much lower rates of multiple births. According to the 2006 Assisted Reproductive Technology Success Rates from the Centers for Disease Control, the live birth rate per cycle for women with ovulatory dysfunction is about 35%. The overall rate of multiple births is about 11%, with generally a lower than 5% rate of triplets of higher-order births. The main risk of IVF for women with PCOS is ovarian hyperstimulation syndrome.

Conclusions

The most effective long-term management of the irregular menstrual bleeding experienced by women with PCOS is implementation of lifestyle change. Weight loss effectively corrects the underlying metabolic and endocrine disorders that predispose these women to dysfunctional bleeding. Pharmacologic intervention with OCPs, progestins, and insulin-sensitizing agents is often warranted. Medical treatments aimed at improving the symptoms of hyperandrogenism and infertility are also effective. Surgical management may be considered for therapy when appropriate.

Selected bibliography

Azziz R, Sanchez L, Knochenhauer E et al. Androgen excess in women: Experience with over 1000 consecutive patients. J Clin Endocrinol Metab 2004;89:453–62.

Azziz R, Carmina E, Dewailly D et al. The Androgen Excess and PCOS Society criteria for the polycystic ovary syndrome: the complete task force report. Fertil Steril 2009;9:456–88.

Barbieri RL, Ryan KJ. Hyperandrogenism, insulin resistance, and acanthosis nigricans syndrome: a common endocrinopathy with distinct pathophysiologic features. Am J Obstet Gynecol 1983;147:90–101.

Centers for Disease Control. 2006 Assisted reproductive technology success rates, national summary and fertility clinic reports, Centers for Disease Control. Atlanta, GA: CDC, 2008.

Costello MF, Shrestha B, Eden J, Sjoblom P, Johnson N, Moran LJ. Insulin-sensitising drugs versus the combined oral contraceptive pill for hirsutism, acne and risk of diabetes, cardiovascular disease, and endometrial cancer in polycystic ovary syndrome. Cochrane Database of Systematic Reviews. 2009, Issue 4. Art. No.: CD005552.

Legro RS, Myers ER, Barnhart HX et al.; Reproductive Medicine Network. Clomiphene, metformin, or both for infertility in the polycystic ovary syndrome. N Engl J Med 2007;356:551–66.

Dahlgren E, Johansson S, Lindstedt G et al. Women with polycystic ovary syndrome wedge resected in 1956 to 1965: a long-term follow-up focusing on natural history and circulating hormones. Fertil Steril 1992;57:505–13.

Farquhar C, Lilford R, Marjoribanks J, Vanderkerchove P. Laparoscopic 'drilling' by diathermy or laser for ovulation induction in anovulatory polycystic ovary syndrome. Cochrane Menstrual Disorders and Subfertility Group Cochrane Database of Systematic Reviews. 2009, Issue 4. Art. No.: CD001122.

Huber-Buchholz MM, Carey CGP, Norman RJ. Restoration of reproductive potential by lifestyle modification in obese polycystic ovary syndrome: role of insulin sensitivity and luteinizing hormone. J Clin Endocrinol Metab 1999;84:1470–4.

Legro RS, Kunselman AR, Dodson WC, Dunaif A. Prevalence and predictors of risk for type 2 diabetes mellitus and impaired glucose tolerance in polycystic ovary syndrome: a prospective, controlled study in 254 affected women. J Clin Endocrinol Metab 1999;84:165–9.

Meldrum DR, Abraham GE. Peripheral and ovarian venous concentrations of various steroid hormones in virilizing ovarian tumors. Obstet Gynecol 1979;53:36–43.

New MI, Lorenzen F, Lerner AJ et al. Genotyping steroid 21-hydroxylase deficiency: hormonal reference data. J Clin Endocrinol Metab 1983;57:320–6.

6

Abnormal Uterine Bleeding due to Anatomic Causes: Diagnosis

Bradley S. Hurst

Carolinas Medical Center, Charlotte, North Carolina, USA

Introduction

Common anatomic causes of abnormal uterine bleeding include uterine fibroids, endometrial polyps, and adenomyosis. Excessive bleeding due to these causes are typically perceived as cyclic, regular, and predictable, but practitioners must realize that many patients do not follow the expected course and may experience occasional episodes of alarming bleeding followed by moderately heavy bleeding in other cycles. Sometimes a woman experiences midcycle bleeding, prolonged bleeding during menses, premenstrual bleeding, or continuous bleeding interspersed with more normal menstrual cycles. In spite of the somewhat confusing variations, the presentation of a woman with abnormal uterine bleeding due to an anatomic abnormality is usually quite different from that of the woman with abnormal uterine bleeding due to ovulatory dysfunction. The diagnosis should be easily and accurately established with a careful history, focused examination, and limited testing. A rational treatment plan can then be individualized for the patient.

Assessing abnormal uterine bleeding due to mechanical/anatomic causes

Before a provider takes a complete history to determine the cause of abnormal genital bleeding during the reproductive years, it helps to consider the major categories within the differential diagnosis. In general, excessive bleeding during the reproductive years may be caused by three common categories and several important but less common categories. The most common causes of abnormal uterine bleeding during the reproductive years are ovulatory dysfunction, pregnancy-related bleeding, and mechanical causes. The provider must consider factors with serious health implications, especially cancer and other neoplasms. Abnormal bleeding may also be a secondary manifestation of conditions such as a hematosalpinx, cervicitis or endometritis, or genital trauma. On occasion, rectal or urinary bleeding may be incorrectly diagnosed as vaginal bleeding.

Avoiding pitfalls in diagnosis and treatment of abnormal uterine bleeding due to mechanical causes

> **✋ CAUTION**
>
> An improperly diagnosed woman with excessive bleeding due to uterine fibroids or endometrial polyps will usually continue to have abnormal bleeding in spite of hormonal intervention and regardless of a change in the type of hormonal contraception. The patient may endure many months of unnecessary suffering and frustration by the time either

Disorders of Menstruation, 1st edition. Edited by Paul B. Marshburn and Bradley S. Hurst.
© 2011 Blackwell Publishing Ltd.

the doctor offers appropriate testing, an accurate diagnosis is made, or the woman seeks a second opinion.

It is important to avoid the "shoot first and ask questions later" approach to abnormal bleeding. Although it is tempting to recommend surgery for all women who present with an anatomic abnormality such as uterine fibroids, it is important to reach a proper diagnosis to avoid ineffective or excessive treatments. For example, a practitioner who treats all irregular bleeding by prescribing hormonal contraception will delay establishing the correct diagnosis and effective treatment of uterine anatomic abnormalities, such as uterine fibroids, sometimes for months. A typical example occurs when a physician reflexively treats a patient who has abnormal uterine bleeding with oral contraceptives. Since abnormal uterine bleeding commonly occurs within the first month or two of hormonal contraceptive use, a patient may be encouraged to continue treatment for two cycles in the hope of improving. However, once hormonal contraception is initiated, it is not unusual for a provider to switch to a different type of hormonal contraception if the patient reports irregular or excessive bleeding.

History

Basic history

Except in emergent situations of life-threatening bleeding, the clinician should always determine the onset of the last normal menstrual period. A good menstrual history will provide valuable information (Table 6.1). Determine the nature of the bleeding: amount, duration, time course, and if there appear to be any exacerbating or relieving factors.

Focused history

With the short list in mind, the practitioner can usually devise a history to identify the underlying cause of abnormal bleeding. Fortunately, the three major categories present distinctly different symptoms, but it is important to consider the subtle features of each.

Table 6.1 Questions for a menstrual history

When did your last period start (full flow)?
How many days does the bleeding last?
How often do you change pads or tampons on the heaviest day of flow? How saturated these are when changed?
How long does the heavy bleeding last?
Are blood clots present? If so, how large are the clots?
Is bleeding present before full flow begins? If so, how much and for how long?
Is cramping present during menses? If so, what measures do you take to relieve the pain (medications—dose, frequency, and duration, heat, bed rest, etc.)? Is there associated nausea, vomiting, or loose stools?
Does this bleeding pattern happen predictably every month?
How long has bleeding been problematic?
Did anything happen around the time the bleeding initially began (completion of pregnancy, onset with menarche, etc)?
Has any testing or treatment been performed in the past?
Do you feel light-headed or tired near the end of your periods?
When did you last have intercourse?
What contraceptive measures are you using?
When did you have your last Pap smear?

The doctor should determine whether the patient has signs or symptoms of ovulatory dysfunction. This is essential to reaching an accurate diagnosis and provide appropriate treatment, since abnormal uterine bleeding due to ovulatory dysfunction can be treated hormonally in most circumstances. Furthermore, finding an anatomic abnormality, such as uterine fibroids, is not proof that the abnormal bleeding is caused by the abnormality. Many women have fibroids, but not all those with fibroids have abnormal bleeding; symptoms will depend on the size, number, and location of the fibroids. Although fibroids do not always cause abnormal bleeding, ovulatory dysfunction is always associated with some menstruation abnormality. Treating irregular bleeding due to ovulatory dysfunction should be the providers' first matter for attention because of the simplicity of the treatment.

First, rule out ovulatory dysfunction by taking a detailed menstrual history. Regular, predictable, bleeding is usually associated with ovulation, even if it is excessive. A woman is almost certainly ovulating if she experiences predictable premenstrual symptoms each cycle such as breast soreness, bloating, emotional lability, or premenstrual cramping. In contrast, irregular bleeding due to anovulation is typically unpredictable, unexpected, and irregular in duration and amount. An anatomic cause of excessive bleeding should be the leading diagnosis for a woman who experiences cyclic, predictable bleeding and any or all of the premenstrual symptoms at intervals associated with normal ovulatory menstrual cycles.

Uterine polyps, fibroids, and adenomyosis are the three most common anatomic causes of abnormal uterine bleeding, and often cause midcycle or intermenstrual bleeding, in addition to excessively heavy or prolonged menses (Table 6.2). Other rarer abnormalities include the presence of an intrauterine device, and endometrial vascular abnormalities such as an arteriovenous malformation or endometrial inflammation (endometritis of various causes). When these conditions cause extramenstrual bleeding, it can be challenging to verify whether the patient is experiencing a component of bleeding due to ovulatory dysfunction. These anatomic defects can cause intermittent, unpredictable bleeding or nearly continuous bleeding. As bleeding becomes more frequent and less predictable, it can be helpful to determine if the woman has recurring cyclic premenstrual-type symptoms, especially if these symptoms are also related to bleeding. Unfortunately, most women who have prolonged, excessive bleeding are unable to separate symptoms into well-defined events, and it

Table 6.2 Differential diagnosis of abnormal uterine bleeding due to anatomic causes

Uterine fibroids
Endometrial or endocervical polyps
Adenomyosis
Intrauterine contraceptive device
"Blood pockets"
Arteriovenous malformation
Hydrosalpinx/hematosalpinx
Uterine or vaginal duplication with partial obstruction
Pregnancy
Endometritis
Endometrial hyperplasia/cancer
Cervical inflammation/cervicitis/cervical dysplasia or cancer
Anatomic plus ovulatory dysfunction

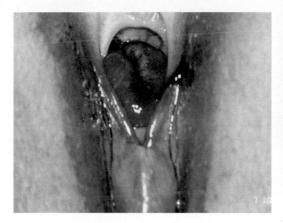

Plate 2.4 Urethral prolapse.

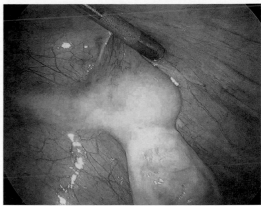

Plate 3.6 Laparoscopic image of nonfunctional rudimentary uterine horns with normal ovaries.

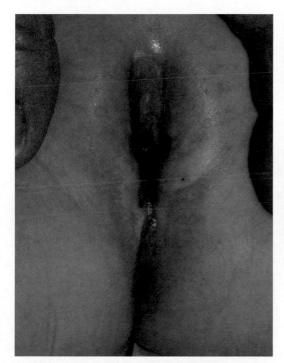

Plate 2.5 Lichen sclerosis et atrophicus.

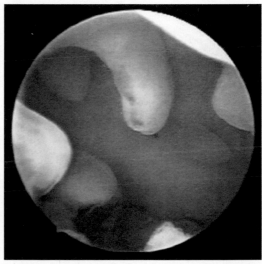

Plate 4.5 Endometrial polyps as visualized by hysteroscopy.

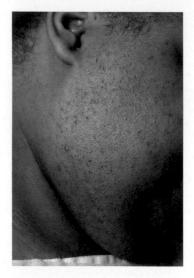

Plate 5.2 Facial hirsutism.

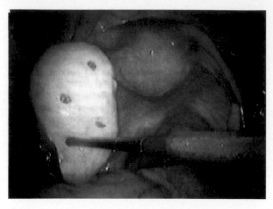

Plate 5.6 Laparoscopic ovarian drilling.

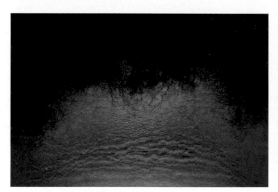

Plate 5.4 Acanthosis nigricans.

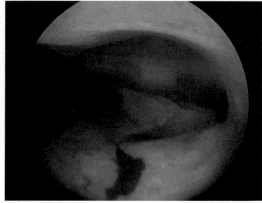

Plate 7.2 Hysteroscopic finding of an endometrial polyp.

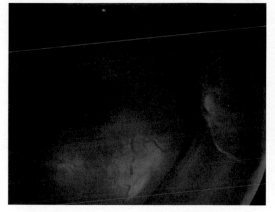

Plate 7.3 Hysteroscopic myomectomy.

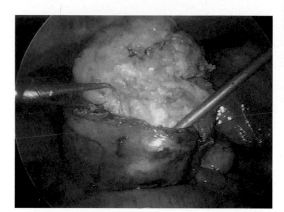

Plate 7.5 Laparoscopic myomectomy initial incision.

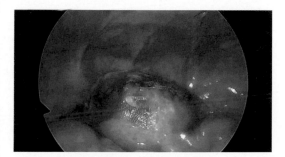

Plate 7.6 Laparoscopic myomectomy placement of an adhesion barrier.

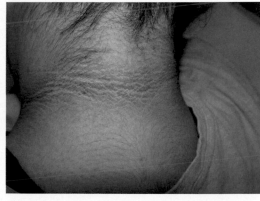

(a)

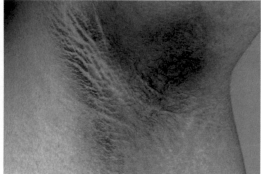

(b)

Plate 8.2 Acanthosis nigricans of (a) the neck and (b) the axilla. Reproduced from (a) www.fromyourdoctor.com and (b) webmd.com.

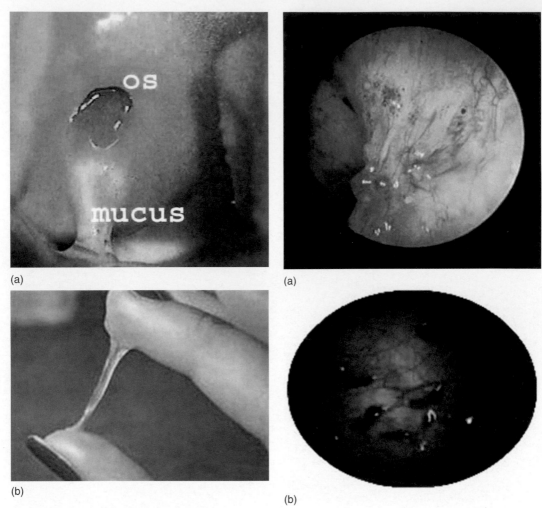

(a)

(b)

Plate 8.4 Estrogenized cervical mucus.
Reproduced from (a) http://infertilitybooks.com
and (b) http://commons.wikimedia.org.

(a)

(b)

Plate 9.3 Appearance of (a) clear and (b) red
endometriosis lesions seen in adolescents.

is necessary to perform additional assessments to correlate the bleeding episodes with ovulatory cycles.

The clinical history of a woman with uterine fibroids varies based on their size, number, and location. Often, a woman presents with a known diagnosis based on a prior clinical evaluation. Most women with endometrial distortion from fibroids will report progressively heavier menses, cramping, and clots, and they may develop intermenstrual bleeding. Curiously, some women describe periods of alternating severity—one normal followed by one heavy period. In most cases, although there may be variation from one cycle to the next, the heaviest bleeding (associated with menstrual bleeding) is cyclic and should be preceded by premenstrual moliminal symptoms. A woman with intracavitary fibroids may also have a history of infertility or poor pregnancy outcomes including miscarriage, bleeding during pregnancy, or postpartum hemorrhage.

Large fibroids that distend the abdomen may cause progressive abdominal bloating, pressure, or pain. The pain may be severe, especially if a fibroid infarcts. Large fibroids can cause uterine enlargement that, in some, protrudes the lower abdomen like an advanced pregnancy. Fibroids that press directly or indirectly against the bladder typically cause urinary frequency, and may cause nocturia and incontinence. Fibroids that compress the rectum inflict constipation or alternating constipation and diarrhea, and can lead to dyspareunia. Rarely, fibroids cause pelvic and back pain associated with dilated ureters and renal calyces from compression of urinary outflow.

Uterine fibroids are most common in women of African descent, but are also found in women of any background, so if symptoms are present they should be considered regardless of race. There are no known factors that cause or prevent fibroids. However, there is a familial tendency for developing fibroids, so it is worthwhile to ask the patient if she has a relative who has required a hysterectomy or other treatment for fibroids. Fibroids are more commonly identified in the late menstrual years, so a woman who presents with typical symptoms of fibroids in her late 30s or 40s should further raise the suspicion of this etiology.

The symptoms of adenomyosis overlap with those of uterine fibroids and include menorrhagia, dysmenorrhea, pelvic pain and midcycle bleeding; the condition typically presents in parous women over 30 years of age. Adenomyosis can be difficult to distinguish from fibroids by clinical history alone, and frequently the conditions coexist. Adenomyosis is a condition that occurs when endometrial tissue is present in the myometrium, or when endometrium is disrupted and dislocated to the myometrium during delivery, a miscarriage, or endometrial instrumentation. However, adenomyosis is also present in some women who lack these historical factors. The tissue is hormonally active and can undergo cyclic proliferation and hemorrhaging similar to the endometrium. The symptoms progress gradually in many women but may progress quickly after a pregnancy is completed. A history of onset of dysmenorrhea and menorrhagia after pregnancy or uterine instrumentation is a clue to the presence of adenomyosis.

A woman with endometrial polyps may present with excessive menstrual bleeding, sometimes associated with clots, dysmenorrhea, and intermenstrual bleeding, but other "bulk" symptoms are not expected. Occasionally, a polyp will prolapse through the cervix, and this can cause postcoital bleeding or a discharge. Polyps can be recurrent. A woman with a history of recurrent menorrhagia and polyps is likely to have recurrent symptoms because of repeated polyps.

The clinical diagnosis may be apparent in some less common causes of abnormal uterine bleeding due to mechanical causes. For example, women sometimes experience increased bleeding and dysmenorrhea after insertion of a copper-containing intrauterine device, but the cause and effect will be evident to the patient and the provider.

Bleeding due to delayed drainage from "pockets"

In other conditions, such as a hematosalpinx, the symptoms are evident but could be overlooked. Bleeding from a hematosalpinx usually occurs throughout the cycle. A retrograde menstrual bleeding into a hydrosalpinx during menses may cause hematosalpinx, followed by drainage from the hematosalpinx into the uterus and discharge from the cervix and vagina for the remainder of the cycle. The midcycle blood tends to be dark and watery, and pain and dyspareunia are common accompanying symptoms.

Similarly, a woman with uterine duplication may experience dysmenorrhea due to the discharge of menstrual blood into the partially obstructed hemivagina, as well as intermenstrual drainage of dark blood as the hemivagina slowly drains. Intercourse may be painful, and causes increased bleeding if it forces the blood to be discharged more rapidly. Symptoms typically begin with menarche. Since many women with uterine or vaginal obstructive anomalies develop endometriosis, the severity of pelvic pain can increase over time.

Prolonged bloody menstrual drainage from a partially enclosed pocket of endometrium in an Asherman syndrome patient is a rare cause of abnormal bleeding. Uterine adhesions occur most often when a woman has experienced a postabortion or postpartum curettage, so verifying the past proximity of onset following curettage or other uterine manipulation is the key to suspecting this possible diagnosis.

The rarely found condition of a uterine or vaginal arteriovenous malformation often has no clearly identifiable historical factors. However, unexpected, unpredictable bleeding in a woman with previously normal menstrual cycles can suggest this condition.

Inflammatory causes

Endometritis is an unusual cause of abnormal uterine bleeding that is caused by a microscopic endometrial alteration. It is most commonly found following completion of a pregnancy, but is also caused by nongravid ascending endometrial infections from various organisms and can even occur in the absence of an identifiable infection.

Risk factors for postpartum or postabortion endometritis include prolonged dilatation of the cervix and retained products of conception. Prolonged cervical dilatation allows ascending infections, and occurs with prolonged rupture of membranes or extended labor. Retained products of conception following a delivery, miscarriage, or termination provide a nest for bacterial colonization and infection. Additionally, bacteria may enter the uterus during a delivery or termination performed under unsanitary conditions or with contaminated instruments. Although irregular bleeding is common in these circumstances, the most obvious clinical symptoms of postpregnancy endometritis are abdominal pain and fever.

Endometritis due to infection or noninfectious inflammation of the endometrium may present with a subtle finding, including a slight increase in the volume or duration of menstrual bleeding, or intermenstrual bleeding. Lower abdominal pain or dyspareunia might occur, but some women have no clinical symptoms whatsoever. Tuberculosis endometritis is a possibility, especially in an infected woman with immunodeficiency, but is rarely the primary symptom. Occasionally, endometritis is diagnosed histologically from an endometrial biopsy in an asymptomatic patient. The pathologist can use special stains to detect plasma cells in endometrial tissue, a pathognomonic histologic sign of endometritis. The clinician, however, must inform the pathologist about the suspicion of endometritis to insure this special staining is performed.

Neoplastic disease and pregnancy

The practitioner must keep potentially life-threatening conditions in mind when interviewing a woman with abnormal uterine bleeding; neoplasia and pregnancy must be considered as part of the differential diagnosis. Neoplastic disorders that cause abnormal uterine bleeding during the reproductive years include cervical dysplasia, cervical carcinoma, endometrial hyperplasia, endometrial carcinoma, leiomyosarcoma, gestational trophoblastic disease, fallopian tubal carcinoma, vulvovaginal carcinoma, and metastatic disease affecting the reproductive organs. Pregnancy-related bleeding may include threatened, complete, or incomplete abortion, ectopic pregnancy, placenta previa, or placental abruption.

Combined abnormalities

The clinical history is much more confusing when a patient has both ovulatory dysfunction and a uterine mechanical abnormality. Women with combined abnormalities may give a history of irregular, unpredictable bleeding with unpredictable amounts and duration, sometimes interspersed with symptoms suggestive of ovulation. When the clinical history is unclear, it is helpful to assess ovulatory function concurrently with uterine abnormalities.

Further complicating the diagnostic dilemma is the pregnant patient with uterine fibroids or known endometrial polyps who has first-trimester bleeding. This patient may experience irregular bleeding prior to conception, and continued abnormal bleeding in early pregnancy, which obscures the proper diagnosis of the pregnancy and the abnormality until further testing confirms both conditions.

Physical examination of a woman with abnormal uterine bleeding

Keen observation and a thorough examination of the patient with abnormal uterine bleeding provide insight into the severity and differential diagnosis of the bleeding, and should be part of the evaluation, but examination rarely provides a definitive diagnosis.

Additional signs and symptoms of severe, life-threatening bleeding include shock, orthostatic hypotension, tachycardia, and pallor, and should be obvious to a women's health provider. The physician must simultaneously assess and stabilize the patient. The process of evaluation and initial treatment of a woman with an anatomic cause of abnormal uterine bleeding is discussed later in the chapter.

General

A woman who has a long history of severe menorrhagia may tolerate severe anemia remarkably well. Nevertheless, a woman with severe menorrhagia-related anemia will often have predictable pallor and pale sclera, especially near the end of each heavy period. She might report light-headedness or fatigue, and could have tachycardia or orthostatic tachycardia and orthostatic hypotension. If the patient is currently bleeding, she may report severe cramping and may experience acute distress from pain, nausea, or vomiting. Blood that saturates clothing is a reliable sign of acute excessive bleeding. Postural vital signs and a description of the woman's general demeanor should be documented whenever a woman presents with heavy bleeding.

Abdominal

An abdominal examination determines whether there is a palpable mass consistent with uterine enlargement, which may occur most often with pregnancy or fibroids. Tenderness should be described, including the presence of guarding or rebound. Usually, since pressure does not affect uterine-related cramping, the pain associated with cramping is not markedly increased by palpation or pressure caused by the passage of clots from anatomic abnormalities such as fibroids, adenomyosis, or polyps. However, the pain is worsened by abdominal palpation when it is due to an infarcting fibroid or by conditions that lead to pelvic inflammation.

Pelvic examination

The pelvic examination provides the examiner with the best information about active bleeding and may provide insight about the possible causes.

Introitus

The extent of bleeding can be assessed by determining how much dried and fresh blood is found on the introitus. Even if bleeding has subsided, a large blood-stained area indicates recent heavy bleeding.

Vagina

The amount of blood found in the vagina during speculum examination should be estimated and described, and the color noted. Bright red blood indicates active bleeding, dark blood indicates "older" blood, and greenish blood has been present for days. Blood clots form in the uterus and pass into the vagina, so the presence of clots confirms uterine bleeding.

Cervix

Examination of the cervix provides the most helpful evaluation of the rate of uterine bleeding. Here again, the red blood provides evidence of active bleeding, and dark blood shows delayed bleeding. Passage of clots through the cervix indicates bleeding into the uterus with a high enough volume for blood to accumulate in the uterine cavity. This is common with uterine polyps, fibroids, and adenomyosis, as well as with first-trimester bleeding. As bleeding increases and decreases in relation to uterine contractions, it is helpful to observe the cervix for a period of time, rather than inspecting quickly. The cervical os may be dilated or effaced if the patient has a prolapsing polyp or fibroid, and sometimes this mass is visibly distending the cervix. Cervical motion tenderness indicates an inflammatory condition, and if adnexal and uterine tenderness accompanies cervical motion tenderness, a preliminary presumptive diagnosis of pelvic inflammatory disease should be considered.

Uterus

During the bimanual examination, the size, position, and shape of the uterus is noted, and tenderness is assessed if present. The uterus is often enlarged and irregular with uterine fibroids due to the distortion from the individual masses. When the uterus is enlarged, the examiner should try to estimate the overall size of the uterus (usually compared to the size of the uterus in at a specific gestational age in weeks). If individual uterine masses are palpated, the size and location of the masses should be carefully assessed and noted. It may be necessary to perform a rectovaginal examination to feel posterior uterine fibroids. The fibroid uterus is usually not tender during the examination unless a fibroid is infarcting.

Adenomyosis can also cause the uterus to enlarge, but a symmetric enlargement due to diffuse adenomyosis is most typical. Occasionally, an adenomyoma forms a distinct nodular mass in the myometrium, which could be confused with a uterine fibroid. Most gynecologists think of the adenomyosis uterus as a big, boggy uterus. Rectovaginal endometriosis, sometimes referred to as adenomyosis, will be identified by palpation of uterosacral nodularity or nodularity in the posterior cul-de-sac, but this type of adenomyosis does not directly cause abnormal uterine bleeding unless myometrial adenomyosis is also present.

The uterus can also be enlarged due to endometrial carcinoma or leiomyosarcoma. However, while practitioners must consider both of these in the differential diagnosis, endometrial carcinoma typically occurs in older women with chronic oligo-ovulation or anovulation, and leiomyosarcoma is most common in postmenopausal women.

The uterine examination will be normal if a woman has endometrial polyps or most other non-inflammatory causes of anatomic uterine bleeding. Tenderness is expected in conditions that cause uterine or endometrial inflammation.

Adnexa

On occasion, examination of the adnexa gives insight into the cause of abnormal uterine bleeding. For example, a firm, nontender adnexal mass is sometimes identified in a woman with a lateral pedunculated uterine fibroid. The fibroid may be fixed if it has a broad-based attachment to the uterus, or mobile if it is pedunculated (attached to the uterus by a "stalk"). The differential diagnosis for a soft, tender, adnexal mass is long, but includes a hydrosalpinx. As noted above, a hydrosalpinx can become blood-filled due to retrograde menstruation, and may cause delayed bleeding as the blood mixes with watery tubal secretions and drains into the uterus.

The provider must be aware of several conditions that limit adnexal examination. If the uterus is larger than the size of a 12-week pregnancy, the adnexa are often dislocated out of the pelvis and usually cannot be palpated. Much to the chagrin of traditionalists who stress the importance of a thorough pelvic examination, ultrasound has enhanced the assessment, and the woman does not experience considerable discomfort as she would during the examination. If a woman feels considerable pain during adnexal palpation, the doctor should use ultrasound instead of subjecting the patient to greater pain by trying to palpate a mass. Finally, although tenderness should always be assessed, the value of an adnexal examination to assess masses is limited in obese women.

Diagnostic tests for abnormal uterine bleeding of suspected anatomic etiology

Laboratory assessment at the initial visit

Initial laboratory testing should follow a common-sense approach and be performed based on the acuity of the presentation. A patient with massive bleeding and signs, or concerns, that she might become hemodynamically unstable is assessed differently from a woman with chronically heavy or prolonged menses. The hemodynamically unstable case will be discussed in another section.

For the woman with typical chronic bleeding abnormalities, a complete blood count should be performed to determine anemia. Chronic excessive bleeding with inadequate iron intake will cause microcytic anemia. Women with anatomic causes of excessive bleeding can adapt remarkably well to severe anemia and may show few symptoms. While a hemodynamically stable patient with severe anemia does not constitute an emergent situation or immediate action, a woman with severe anemia has little reserve, and an efficient evaluation and appropriate treatment plan need to be implemented. For a woman with chronically heavy bleeding, the ideal time to determine anemia is during or immediately after the heaviest days of flow.

Human chorionic gonadotropin

Unless the provider is certain that the patient is not pregnant, a pregnancy test should be a routine part of the evaluation for reproductive-age women. It is important to test for pregnancy for several reasons. For example, during the evaluation of abnormal bleeding, it may be necessary to perform tests that include radiographs, such as a hysterosalpingogram (HSG), or that use uterine instrumentation, such as saline infusion sonohysterography (SIS). A pregnancy can be damaged by either procedure, so a test is a simple, accurate, inexpensive way to avoid harming the fetus. Furthermore, many pregnancy-related conditions such as ectopic pregnancy, hematoma, or miscarriage sometimes cause heavy bleeding, and one must consider these conditions in the differential diagnosis. No contraceptive is 100% effective, and the patient may be unwilling to admit to recent intercourse, or may be unexpectedly pregnant. Obtaining a negative serum result as an initial part of the evaluation excludes these conditions from the differential diagnosis.

Serum human chorionic gonadotropin (hCG) tests are more sensitive than urine tests. Most urine tests detect hCG levels of approximately 25 IU/mL (IU/mL), whereas most serum assays measure levels above 5 IU/mL, although there is considerable variation in serum hCG levels between different laboratories, depending on the assay used. To put these numbers in context, a pregnant woman's hCG levels are approximately 25–100 IU/mL on the first day she misses a period, 2 weeks after ovulation. With a normal pregnancy, the quantitative hCG level typically doubles in early pregnancy, and an increase of 67% or more is in the normal range. The differences between tests mean that a serum test is likely to be positive a few days earlier than a urine test. In most cases, the convenience and low cost of a urine test outweighs the slightly inferior sensitivity of the serum test. However, when the urine pregnancy test is positive for a woman with irregular bleeding, it is important to obtain a serum hCG level, as discussed in other chapters.

At least two other initial tests should be considered at the time of the initial evaluation: a Papanicolau smear and cervical screening for gonorrhea and *Chlamydia*. Unfortunately, the sensitivity of the Papanicolau smear is reduced in a woman with active menstrual bleeding, but it is important to exclude cervical dysplasia or carcinoma by obtaining cervical cytology, unless a negative test was obtained within the recommended screening interval: 2 years for women in their 20s, and every 3 years beginning age 30. If the smear is abnormal, appropriate testing must be performed, which may include HIV screening, colposcopy, or other tests (outlined elsewhere).

Similarly, screening for gonorrhea and chlamydia is advisable for young sexually active women. Among females, half of all chlamydia cases are identified in girls from age 15 to 19, and 33% occur in women between 20 and 24, according to statistics from the Centers for Diseases Control. By some estimates, approximately 10% of sexually active teenage girls are carriers of *Chlamydia*. Chlamydia and gonorrhea may be asymptomatic, but both can cause cervicitis and irregular bleeding. More importantly, ascending infections may cause salpingitis and result in pelvic inflammatory disease, infertility, and increased risk for ectopic pregnancy.

The Centers for Diseases Control recommend that all sexually active women should be screened annually for chlamydia and gonorrhea until age 25, and women over 25 should be screened when they have a new or multiple sexual partners. In the past, cervical cultures were required to diagnose these infections, but the standard screening in the United States today uses specific DNA probes. Screening can be done by urine or by cervical swab, in combination with liquid Papanicolau tests. If the practitioner is uncertain about whether or not to screen, it is best to err on the side of caution and perform the test.

Determining ovulatory status when history is not conclusive

> ★ TIPS & TRICKS
>
> Evidence of heavy or irregular bleeding in the presence of regular ovulation cycles almost always indicates the presence of an anatomic etiology such as polyps, fibroids, or adenomyosis. Often, a simple history will suffice to confirm ovulation, and the practitioner can immediately begin testing to identify the underlying anatomic abnormality.

In some cases with prolonged, excessive bleeding, it is not clear whether the bleeding is caused by an anatomic abnormality associated with ovulatory cycles or by chronic anovulation. This is crucial to determine, since most causes of abnormal uterine bleeding due to ovulatory dysfunction can be treated hormonally, and most anatomic causes require surgical intervention to relieve symptoms. Several simple, inexpensive tests include and a menstrual calendar and a basal body temperature (BBT) chart, targeted or weekly progesterone levels, or an endometrial biopsy, and can provide insight in these complex cases. A doctor can usually reach a determination within a month of the initial consultation visit.

Menstrual calendar

When kept properly, a menstrual calendar provides a record of each daily occurrence and the severity of bleeding over a certain period, usually at least 1 month. It is straightforward and easy for the patient and the provider as it simply involves a daily recording of the amount of bleeding, if any. A small checkbook calendar with the dates "encoded" to describe the bleeding can be adequate. One method is to underline a day of spotting, circle a day of "full" flow, and circle and fill in days of heavy flow. Color-coding can also be used. The appeal of this approach is the simplicity and ready availability of a calendar, but it is limited in determining whether bleeding is related to ovulatory dysfunction or an anatomic abnormality, especially in a patient who has non-cyclic bleeding.

Basal body temperature

BBT charting has a clear advantage over keeping a menstrual calendar in that it allows the provider to determine the relation of bleeding to ovulation. BBT recording relies on the principle that the rise in progesterone levels that occurs after ovulation increases the BBT. Before ovulation, most women have a "basal" body temperature less than 98°F (36.7°C). After ovulation, temperature is usually 98°F or higher. The temperature typically falls a day or two before the onset of menses, but temperature patterns are not reliable predictors of ovulation. Because of this limitation, BBT is not a very helpful test for fertility and has become an underused tool, especially in evaluating women with abnormal bleeding. BBT monitoring has the great advantage that the only costs are a thermometer and paper, and is extremely informative to the enlightened provider.

In order to keep an accurate BBT chart, the patient must be willing and able to record her temperature before getting out of bed when she wakes each morning. A rapid digital oral thermometer is the easiest to use. The easier BBT charting is, the more compliant the patient will probably be. Special BBT thermometers are unnecessary. The body temperature changes once the patient has got out of bed, so if a woman forgets it is best to leave the daily temperature blank rather than record an erroneous or misleading measurement. BBT also varies if the time of waking varies considerably from day to day, so odd-hour shift workers or women who travel frequently to different time zones are not ideal candidates for BBT. Fever from illness or oral temperature change due to beverage consumption can confound BBT measurements, and patients should be educated about these pitfalls. Calendars for logging BBT are available online, but simple graph paper may be used, as well with temperature range listed from 96 to 99 °F (35.5 to 37.2 °C).

In addition to recording daily temperature, a woman with abnormal uterine bleeding should document the amount of bleeding she experiences each day. Simple codes are best: "S" for spotting, "L" for light bleeding, "M" for moderate bleeding, "H" for heavy, "X" for excessive, with a notation of "C" for clots, if present. It is also helpful to keep a recording of intercourse, since cervicitis, cervical polyps, dysplasia, or vaginal or vulvar lesions can all be associated with postcoital bleeding.

Once a patient with abnormal bleeding has tracked her BBT for 1–3 months, the provider can use the charts to determine if she is ovulating (indicated by a persistent temperature rise, usually 98 °F or higher, for at least 1 week). If ovulation presents, bleeding should occur after the temperature falls. If bleeding occurs throughout the cycle in a woman with a biphasic BBT, the provider can be almost certain that the bleeding is due to an anatomic abnormality and not to ovulatory dysfunction (Figure 6.1). In this circumstance, imaging with SIS is the most informative test.

When bleeding occurs after a temperature fall (indicating menstrual bleeding) and "extramenstrual" bleeding happens primarily after intercourse, a cervical, vaginal, or vulvar cause is the most likely cause. A careful re-examination of these structures, a Papanicolaou smear if not previously done, and screening for gonorrhea, *Chlamydia*, and *Trichomonas* should be performed if indicated by physical findings. If the temperature is monophasic, or variable with no temperature shift, the bleeding is most likely caused by ovulatory dysfunction. An endometrial biopsy is appropriate if the patient is in an age group that indicates a risk for endometrial hyperplasia or endometrial cancer. If she is in a low-risk age group, hormonal management and intermittent progestin therapy or hormonal contraception is appropriate.

Serum progesterone levels

For some women with unclear symptoms of ovulation, it may not be practical to obtain a BBT recording. Laboratory testing may be needed in these cases. The simplest method is obtaining a serum progesterone during the expected luteal phase, based on typical premenstrual symptoms. Ovulation is confirmed in most laboratories if the progesterone level is 2 ng/mL or higher. This is lower than the "ideal" peak progesterone level of 8–12 ng/mL that is sometimes associated with a luteal phase insufficiency, as the lower levels indicate that ovulation has not occurred. It is not a measure of the "quality" of the corpus luteum function. Progesterone levels increase after ovulation and decline before menses. Therefore, with elevation above 2 ng/mL but relatively low levels, menses can be expected within a few days if progesterone levels are falling, or in 10–14 days if levels are rising in the postovulatory interval. If progesterone levels are elevated, bleeding that occurs at about the expected time based on the progesterone level is likely to be menstrual bleeding; bleeding at other times is likely due to an anatomic abnormality.

Progesterone levels are low, less than 2 ng/mL, before ovulation, so a low progesterone level does not confirm ovulatory dysfunction on one occasion. Since the follicular phase of the menstrual cycle is approximately 14 days and can vary from 11 to 21 days in women whose cycles range from 25 to 35 days, it may be necessary to measure progesterone levels weekly for up to three consecutive weeks to determine whether ovulation occurs in association with irregular bleeding. Once the progesterone level is above 2 ng/mL, additional measurements are not needed. The provider simply compares the onset and duration of bleeding with the expected time of menses. Again, if bleeding occurs any time other than the time of expected menses in an ovulatory woman, or if menstrual bleeding is excessive, it is almost certain that an anatomic abnormality is the cause. If the patient has three consecutive weekly progesterone levels less than 2 ng/mL, ovulatory dysfunction is the likely cause of abnormal bleeding, especially if the patient has bled throughout the monitored interval.

Cycle	1	2	3	4	5	6	7	8	9	10	11	12	13	14	15	16	17	18	19	20	21	22	23	24	24	26	27	28	29	30	31	32
Date (September)	5	6	7	8	9	10	11	12	13	14	15	16	17	18	19	20	21	22	23	24	25	26	27	28	29	30	Oct 1	2	3	4	5	6
Bleeding	H	C	C	C	H	M	H	S	S	S	S	L	M	H	S	S	S		S	S	S	M	S	S	S	L	M	M	H	C	C	C
99																																
.9																													x			
.8																															x	x
.7																														x		
.6																														x		
.5															x																	
.4																										x						
.3																	x		x		x		x		x		x					
.2																		x		x		x		x				x				
.1																																
98																																
.9																x																
.8										x																						
.7					x							x																				
.6		x				x																										
.5	x							x	x		x				x																	
.4			x										x																			
.3				x										x																		
.2																																
.1																																
97																																
.9																																

Figure 6.1 Basal body temperature chart showing a biphasic temperature before and after ovulation, with bleeding episodes marked. This shows evidence of ovulation and intermenstrual bleeding, consistent with an anatomic cause. S, spotting; L, light; M, moderate; C, clots/heavy; empty squares, no bleeding.

Endometrial biopsy

An endometrial biopsy is a screening test for endometrial hyperplasia and endometrial carcinoma in a woman with abnormal uterine bleeding, but information obtained during this biopsy can sometimes help the clinician confirm ovulation. After ovulation, the endometrium matures in a predictable sequence until menses occurs, allowing the postovulatory interval to be "dated," and the onset of menstrual bleeding can be predicted. Therefore, if an endometrial biopsy shows "secretory" changes, confirming that ovulation has occurred, an anatomic cause is likely. However, just as a single low progesterone result does not identify the status of ovulatory dysfunction, the finding of a "proliferative" pattern on endometrial biopsy does not prove the absence of ovulation.

Histologic patterns may be identified by endometrial biopsy. A hemorrhagic or disorganized endometrium is common when a woman is bleeding. On other occasions, inflammation may be present, but this finding is not diagnostic: it can occur with an anatomic abnormality, can help diagnose endometritis, or may be an impertinent finding. Use of an endometrial biopsy to assess cancer or life-threatening uterine bleeding is addressed in other chapters.

Imaging studies to evaluate abnormal uterine bleeding with suspected anatomic etiology

Four mainstay imaging tests are performed for women with abnormal uterine bleeding and a suspected anatomic abnormality: ultrasonography, SIS, HSG, and magnetic resonance imaging (MRI) (Table 6.3). It is essential for the provider to understand the information that is provided by these tests, and the advantages and limitations of each test in determining the most informative and cost-effective approach for each patient, depending on her symptoms, physical findings, and objectives. A "one size fits all" approach to testing is inappropriate. It is equally unsuitable to order expensive tests unless the results establish a rational treatment plan.

Ultrasonography

Ultrasonography evaluates almost all women with suspected anatomic abnormalities, unless the diagnosis and optimal treatment are apparent based on history and examination. Vaginal ultrasound examination usually provides better image quality than abdominal ultrasound, but

Table 6.3 Evaluation of anatomic abnormal uterine bleeding

History
Examination
Testing
Ultrasound
Saline sonography
Magnetic resonance imaging
Laboratory studies
Complete blood count
If the woman desires pregnancy: ovarian reserve testing, semen analysis, possible hysterosalpingography
Endometrial biopsy if cancer is suspected

both methods might be necessary if the uterus is markedly enlarged, as with uterine fibroids, or if the patient is unwilling or unable to undergo vaginal ultrasonography. Abdominal ultrasound examination is also needed if the ovaries are not seen by vaginal ultrasound. Overlying bowel or bowel gas limits the visualization of the uterus and ovaries; therefore abdominal ultrasound for gynecologic indications should be done with the bladder full enough to cover the uterus and form a "window" for the examination. Vaginal probe ultrasound studies are usually performed with an empty bladder for patient comfort.

Careful examination of the endometrium, myometrium, and ovaries is needed to assess anatomic abnormalities, but an understanding of the physiologic and anatomic changes that occur during the menstrual cycle provides greater insight into the underlying cause of abnormal uterine bleeding. First, consider that the endometrium is typically thin (less than 6 mm) during menses and then grows as estradiol increases, corresponding to growth of a preovulatory follicle during the follicular phase of the menstrual cycle. Throughout menses, the ovaries are typically inactive with no hormone-producing cyst, although a residual corpus luteum cyst might be identified.

As the endometrium thickens in the preovulatory interval, it will often form a "triple stripe" or trilaminar layer (Figure 6.2) approximately 7–14 mm thick, and the endometrial develop-

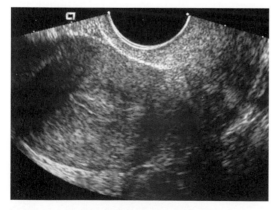

Figure 6.2 Ultrasound with a trilaminar pattern and a hyperechoic defect suggestive of a polyp or submucous myoma.

ment corresponds to growth of the preovulatory follicle, which reaches a maximal diameter of 20–30 mm before ovulation. Endometrial polyps or submucous myomas are easily seen with the triple stripe pattern (Figure 6.2), and the absence of endometrial distortion or continuity of the "white line" (specular reflection) in a trilaminar endometrium makes these abnormalities unlikely. After ovulation, the endometrium becomes more homogeneously echogenic or develops a "white" pattern, and this corresponds to formation of a corpus luteum cyst, an irregular cystic mass in the ovary, often with a "marbling" pattern. Endometrial distortion is difficult to assess with a homogeneous endometrial pattern.

This simple understanding of ultrasound assessment of ovulatory physiology can help the provider reach an accurate diagnosis, especially when the ultrasound findings correspond to the pattern of bleeding. For example, ultrasound findings of a thin endometrium and an ovary with no cyst or follicle larger than 10 mm in a woman who experiences extremely heavy bleeding is consistent with menstrual bleeding. Finding a trilaminar endometrium of 8 mm and a corresponding ovarian follicle of 18 mm indicates that the patient is preovulatory, and bleeding that occurs around the time of ovulation is likely due to an anatomic cause, even if a polyp or fibroid is not apparent. Visualization of a 10 mm white endometrium with an irregular hemorrhagic ovarian cyst in a woman who is bleeding should make the physician suspect premenstrual bleeding due to an anatomic abnormality.

On the other hand, a woman who experiences unpredictable, irregular bleeding and has a 12 mm endometrium and has a large number of follicles less than 10 mm in each ovary likely has bleeding due to ovulatory dysfunction, possibly related to polycystic ovarian disease. Alternatively, a thin endometrium and multiple small follicles and irregular bleeding are probably related to a chronic hypoestrogenic ovulatory dysfunction.

Endometrial abnormalities are most obvious when the endometrium has a trilaminar pattern, but one can see subtle abnormalities with careful examination in some circumstances of endometrial polyps or fibroids. For example, a polyp may have a slightly different echogenic pattern from the remainder of the endometrium, or may be surrounded by a small amount of fluid. The physician must be careful not to be misled by the presence of an endometrial blood clot as it can have the same appearance as a polyp. A submucous myoma may also be difficult to identify by ultrasound, especially if the echogenic pattern of the fibroid is similar to the pattern of the surrounding endometrium. Similar to polyps, fibroids in the endometrial cavity are most readily seen by ultrasonography in the preovulatory interval, and most difficult to identify when the endometrium develops a homogeneous pattern after ovulation.

Uterine fibroids or adenomyosis can be found by ultrasound examination of the myometrium in some cases of abnormal uterine bleeding, but these conditions might exist even if the ultrasound is normal. Uterine fibroids may appear different with ultrasound, depending on its characteristics. For example, a calcified myoma has a bright echogenic pattern and distortion or "artifact" beyond the mass (Figure 6.3). Although calcified fibroids are easy to identify, distortion that occurs beyond the myoma may "hide" other fibroids. Uterine fibroids are sometimes visible as "hypoechogenic" oval masses in the myometrium or, less often, have the same echogenic pattern as the surrounding myometrium. More subtle findings of uterine fibroids may be found by identifying deflection of the endometrial or the serosal surface of the uterus (Figure 6.4). These subtle

findings must be interpreted with caution, since normal physiologic contractions of the myometrium can be confused with an intramural fibroid. If a subtle abnormality is suspected, the ultrasonographer should reassess the area of interest after a few minutes to allow a contracted area to change.

Adenomyosis can have several appearances on ultrasound, and it may be confusing to establish the diagnosis. To make it even more confusing, hormonal changes might cause adenomyosis to appear differently throughout the cycle, since the response of adenomyosis is similar to the normal endometrial response. As a result, these lesions may be hyperechoic, hypoechoic, or mixed. They can enlarge or shrink in a matter of days, depending on the hormonal response. Adenomyosis forms nodular masses within the myometrium and can be readily identified by ultrasound. It can also be a more diffuse process that affects large segments of the myometrium, resulting in a subtle uterine enlargement. Adenomyosis and uterine fibroids sometimes have a remarkably similar appearance with ultrasound, and both conditions can present in the same patient. Color Doppler studies are helpful to distinguish uterine fibroids from adenomyosis, since vascular flow is peripheral with fibroids, and more homogeneously affects adenomyosis lesions.

The discovery of ovarian abnormalities might in some circumstances influence care for anatomic abnormal uterine bleeding. For example, when an ovarian cyst that requires surgery is identified, such as an endometrioma, a benign cystic teratoma, or a complex ovarian cyst

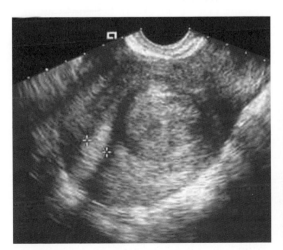

Figure 6.3 Ultrasound with calcified uterine fibroid.

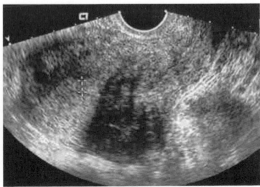

Figure 6.4 Ultrasound with subserosal myoma.

suspicious for neoplasm, nonsurgical options are less appropriate. If ovarian cancer is suspected based on ultrasonographic characteristics of the ovarian mass, including Doppler flow studies and vascular resistance patterns, hysterectomy and bilateral ovarian removal may be appropriate. Another situation where surgery is appropriate is finding a hydrosalpinx in an infertile woman. A visible hydrosalpinx reduces live birth rates from in vitro fertilization (IVF) by approximately 50%, and studies have shown that salpingectomy improves outcomes for IVF and natural conception as long as the contralateral tube is normal. These conditions do not directly cause abnormal uterine bleeding, but the findings make surgery the most appropriate option.

In rare circumstances, delayed drainage of a hematosalpinx or other "pockets" of blood that collect in the uterus or vagina cause abnormal bleeding. Bleeding in these cases is likely associated with dark watery blood between menses. Pelvic pain and dyspareunia are expected when a hematosalpinx is present. Retrograde menstruation into a hydrosalpinx causes the hematosalpinx, and the abnormal bleeding results from the delayed drainage of fluid from the tube into the uterus. Ultrasound examination may reveal a hydrosalpinx—an elongated cystic mass with incomplete septations usually adjacent to the ovary. A hematosalpinx is identified by hemorrhagic echogenic changes within a hydrosalpinx. If pressure from the vaginal ultrasound probe compresses the hydrosalpinx, the patient can experience pain during the examination and an increase in watery bleeding afterwards.

Ultrasound may be helpful in identifying congenital uterine and vaginal anomalies that result in partial obstruction and delayed drainage. One example would be a woman with a unicornuate uterus and an active müllerian remnant, or anlagen, in which the anlagen drains into the uterus via a small communicating opening. In this case, ultrasound clearly identifies the more normal unicornuate uterus and the contralateral anlagen. If present, blood should be readily evident by ultrasound in the anlagen, confirming the diagnosis.

Since most sonographers place the probe in the upper vagina in order to see the uterus, vaginal blood pockets can be difficult or impossible to see with normal vaginal probe ultrasound techniques, but uterine anomalies are likely present and should raise suspicion of a vaginal etiology. Vaginal "pockets" with drainage often occur in women with cervical and uterine duplication, such as a didelphic uterus, a septate uterus with two cervical ostia, or a bicornuate bicollis uterus (a double uterus joined at the cervix with cervical duplication). These conditions are associated with vaginal duplication, and if one hemivagina is partially obstructed, blood will collect in the vagina pouch. Progressively severe pain increases with each menses near menarche if there is complete obstruction of the hemivagina due to vaginal distention from accumulating blood, but delayed and prolonged bleeding is more typical of a patient with communication between the partially obstructed hemivagina and the "normal" vagina.

Since a vaginal probe is not usually used in a position to assess the vagina, vaginal anomalies are likely to be compressed and drained by placement of the vaginal probe, or be completely overlooked during assessment of the cervix, uterus, and adnexa. Abdominal probe ultrasounds are invaluable toward reaching an initial diagnosis of this condition. A fluid-filled mass should be evident inferior to the cervix with abdominal ultrasound, and this mass may be palpable on vaginal or rectal examination.

Other abnormalities found during examination of a woman with anatomic abnormal uterine bleeding may be difficult to categorize initially, but pursuing these findings can lead to a correct diagnosis. For example, if the ultrasound examination reveals endometrial calcifications, the etiology of the calcifications is usually unclear, and may be initially uncertain if the abnormality contributes to abnormal bleeding. Further evaluation is required, and in this circumstance a hysteroscopy and focused biopsy or removal of the calcified area is the most efficient approach. Pursuing this can identify a calcified polyp or fibroid, calcified products of conception, calcified endometrium due to chronic inflammatory conditions, or unexplained calcifications completely unrelated to the bleeding. On one occasion, hysteroscopic removal of a calcified endometrial mass revealed "fetal bone" when evaluated.

A uterine or cervical arteriovenous malformation can cause massive bleeding, and ultrasound may be normal or show a subtle difference in the echogenic pattern of the endometrium or the myometrium. The practitioner should assess subtle abnormalities in either the myometrium or endometrium of a woman with undiagnosed abnormal bleeding with color Doppler studies. A vascular abnormality cannot be definitively diagnosed with Doppler, but detection of much greater than expected blood flow in a small lesion would certainly raise suspicion of a vascular abnormality, and additional diagnostic evaluation with MRI can lead to the correct diagnosis.

Saline infusion sonohysterography

SIS should be performed any time management would be changed if an intracavitary abnormality were identified. For example, if bleeding due to a polyp or submucous myoma is suspected but not proven by history and ultrasound examination, and a conservative medical or surgical option is considered, SIS can provide invaluable information. On the other hand, if hysterectomy is most appropriate and identification of a polyp or submucous myoma would not change care, SIS is not warranted.

SIS requires the placement of an intracervical catheter to instill saline into the uterus while performing transvaginal sonography. Traditional sonography does not easily differentiate fibrous and muscular fibroid tissue from surrounding fibrous and muscular myometrium, but it is a very powerful and sensitive tool in identifying the contrast between solid tissue and fluid. Intracavitary abnormalities are highlighted by this technique. We use SIS after first performing a comprehensive transvaginal ultrasound examination. After the vaginal probe has been removed, a speculum is placed into the vagina, with the cervix visualized and ideally positioned in the center of the speculum blades. The cervix is cleaned with betadine or a similar agent, and a catheter is passed through the cervix into the uterus. The endometrial cavity is imaged longitudinally from one side to the other, and then transversely from the top of the cavity to the cervix.

> ★ **TIPS & TRICKS**
>
> We use a thin, long, semirigid insemination catheter, like a Shepherd or a Soule catheter. A small commercially available uterine balloon-tipped catheter intended for saline infusion sonohysterography is convenient and is used by many, but a thin pediatric Foley catheter may be used. Once the catheter has been set, care is taken to avoid pulling the catheter out while the speculum is removed. The vaginal probe is placed, and the cavity visualized while the smallest amount of fluid is slowly instilled—slow instillation minimizes uterine cramping. Unless the cervix is dilated, 5–20 mL of saline is a sufficient volume for the entire study.

A normal cavity has a "tear" shape. Polyps and submucous myomas project completely into the endometrial cavity (Figure 6.5). It may be difficult to differentiate between these two defects, although polyps are more likely to move with the flow of saline, and very small elongated defects are also more likely to be polyps (Figure 6.6). A sessile myoma—a fibroid that extends from the myometrium into the endometrium—can be easily identified by SIS, with the fibroid penetrating into the cavity (Figure 6.7). Rarely, an adenomyosis nodule extends from the myometrium into the endometrial cavity and is confused with a sessile myoma. If adenomyosis is suspected, it is helpful to inspect the lesion with color flow Doppler ultrasonography: adenomyosis will

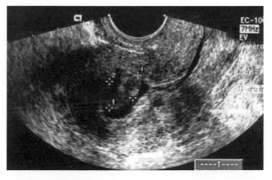

Figure 6.5 Saline infusion sonohysterography showing a submucous myoma.

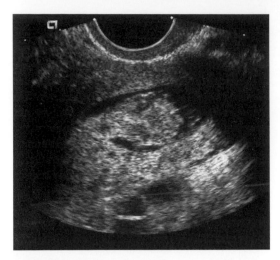

Figure 6.6 Saline infusion sonohysterography showing an elongated polyp.

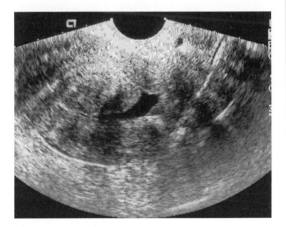

Figure 6.7 Saline infusion sonohysterography showing a sessile myoma.

show flow through the entire mass, whereas flow is typically at the periphery of a fibroid.

As useful as SIS is to identify endometrial abnormalities, it is not an accurate test to identify intracervical abnormalities. In almost all techniques used for SIS, the catheter is placed well into the cervix or completely into the uterine cavity. As a result, the SIS catheter may be placed beyond a cervical polyp or fibroid. Once the uterine cavity has been completely assessed with ultrasound during SIS, if no abnormality is identified the catheter should ideally be slowly removed while continuing to inject saline and

continuing to visualize the ultrasound image. Even if the catheter is placed below the defect and saline infused, the limited distensibility of the cervix may limit visualization. If no abnormality has been identified by ultrasound or SIS in a woman with a suspected anatomic etiology, the differential diagnosis should still include a cervical abnormality such as a polyp, cervicitis, or dysplasia or carcinoma, or a uterine abnormality including adenomyosis or endometritis.

✋ CAUTION

Since a catheter is introduced into the uterine cavity, saline infusion sonohysterography (SIS) should never be performed when pregnancy is suspected. SIS should be performed early in the menstrual cycle, after bleeding stops and before ovulation. After ovulation, the endometrium is irregular and endometrial fragments may be dislodged by the catheter, giving a false-positive result by showing irregular tissue in the uterine cavity. If timing is uncertain due to irregular bleeding, a serum progesterone level and pregnancy test can be performed on the day of or the day before the procedure. A progesterone level less than 2 ng/mL indicates a preovulatory state, and SIS can be performed without risk to an early pregnancy. Alternatively, SIS can be performed at any time except during withdrawal bleeding for a woman using hormonal contraception. SIS can also be performed after suppression with a gonadotropin-releasing hormone agonist.

SIS should never be performed when a pelvic infection is suspected, since the procedure may exacerbate the infection. Antibiotic prophylaxis is not indicated for SIS, but if a hydrosalpinx is identified, broad-spectrum antibiotics, such a doxycycline 100 mg twice daily for 10 days, should be prescribed to prevent "reactivation" of the infection. Finally, although cramping is usually minimal and well tolerated, use of ibuprofen 600 mg orally approximately 30–60 minutes before the procedure will make some patients more comfortable.

Three- and four-dimensional sonography

Three- and four-dimensional sonography is helpful in providing information to reconstruct an image of a solid–fluid interface, but adds little to the diagnosis beyond the two-dimensional assessment of the uterus and SIS imaging of the endometrium. One exception to this is a woman who has several intrauterine abnormalities identified during SIS, since three-dimensional imaging provides a more complete image of the endometrial cavity than single-plane imaging. In practice, however, this advantage in providing slightly more insight into an endometrium with multiple defects is essentially negated during treatments such as hysteroscopy or hysterectomy, since all endometrial lesions should be identified and removed. A second circumstance in which three-dimensional SIS is helpful is for a patient who has rapid leakage of fluid and loss of uterine distention. The three-dimensional scan can capture the image before the fluid escapes the cavity, and allows for analysis.

Hysterosalpingogram

The HSG is an underused diagnostic test for a woman with abnormal uterine bleeding. It provides valuable information for a woman who is interested in future fertility: assessment of tubal patency. A well-performed HSG can identify many abnormalities in the uterine cavity that cause abnormal uterine bleeding, with several advantages and disadvantages compared to SIS. Rarely are both HSG and SIS necessary, and in order to obtain the most diagnostic information in a cost-effective manner, the provider must decide which test is best for the patient.

The most obvious role for HSG is supplying diagnostic information about the uterine cavity and fallopian tubes of an infertile woman, even if abnormal bleeding is not a problem. The HSG is even more important for an infertile woman with abnormal uterine bleeding. Some anatomic abnormalities, including polyps or fibroids, may cause mechanical obstruction of the proximal fallopian tube. The effect of treatment on tubal patency and preservation or enhancement of fertility must be considered. For example, if hysteroscopic loop resection of a fibroid is planned, the relationship of the fibroid to the tubal ostium should be taken into account to avoid damage that causes permanent tubal occlusion. In another example, if the tube is patent but clearly deviated by an intramural myoma and myomectomy is planned, the surgeon needs to be careful to approach the fibroid with the goal of removal and preserving the fallopian tube.

When used with optimal technique, the HSG provides an image of the cervix, the uterine cavity, and the fallopian tubes. The HSG can be performed by several catheter systems to fill the uterus with contrast, including the balloon uterine infusion catheter noted above, a more traditional "acorn" catheter, or a suction catheter. Of these three systems, the authors prefer the acorn and suction catheters to assess the uterine cavity for a woman with abnormal bleeding, since these are placed in the lower cervix and cervical abnormalities can be identified in addition to uterine defects. By comparison, the intrauterine balloon catheter is used by placing the catheter in the uterus, holding it in place by inflating a balloon, and then injecting contrast into the cavity. Inflating the balloon catheter in the uterus can obscure uterine abnormities such as polyps or fibroids, and since the catheter is placed above the cervix, imaging of the cervix is limited.

The uterus must be filled with the uterine cavity parallel to the imaging system in order to detect subtle defects. In order to accomplish this "parallel" imaging for a uterus that is anteverted or retroflexed, it is necessary to obtain traction of the cervix as contrast is slowly filling the cervix and uterus. Traction is accomplished by pulling a cervical tenaculum or the suction device towards the introitus during examination. As this causes cramping, the traction can be stopped after early images of filling of the uterus have been obtained. Cramping is minimized by preprocedural administration of ibuprofen 600–800 mg 30–60 minutes before the procedure. Occasionally, the uterus is so sharply anteverted or retroflexed that traction causes too much discomfort. When this is the case, the provider can push the cervix away from the introitus to completely invert the uterus. The uterine images should always show an elongated uterine cavity that tapers into the lower uterine segment, and not two triangles reflecting the upper uterus and the lower uterine segment. A "two-triangle" image indicates suboptimal assessment of the uterine cavity. Lateral images may help identify an asymmetric flexion of the uterine cavity caused by a large anterior or posterior submucous lesion.

Two simple but important points must be made about optimal performance of HSG: no air or bubbles should be present anywhere within the catheter system, and the uterus should be filled slowly under constant fluoroscopic visualization. Air bubbles can be mistaken for anatomic filling defects of the cavity, or may obscure the image of actual defects. If air bubbles are suspected, they will usually follow the flow of contrast and migrate to the upper uterus during the examination, so a filling defect that moves is almost certainly an air bubble. If the provider is still unsure, the patient should roll slightly to the right, left, or both sides, and additional images should be obtained. Air bubbles will move with position changes, whereas polyps and fibroids will not. The uterus should be filled slowly, since rapid filling causes cramping, and overdistension of the cavity can obscure subtle abnormalities. Fluoroscopy continuously monitors the procedure, and targeted permanent images are captured at key moments during the examination, including early fill of the uterus, tubal fill, and tubal spill.

The HSG is one of the most sensitive imaging tests in identifying a cervical polyp. A cervical polyp is visualized as a filling defect within the cervix and may be completely surrounded by contrast, or may be seen as a filling defect arising from a lateral wall of the cervix (Figure 6.8). If a cervical polyp is seen in a woman with abnormal bleeding, and the HSG is otherwise normal, it is possible to remove the polyp and correct the bleeding in an office setting by performing a cervical curettage.

A submucous myoma is usually indistinguishable from a polyp during the HSG. Both conditions appear as an immobile globular filling defect in the uterine cavity. As with a cervical polyp, a polyp or fibroid may be completely surrounded by contrast, or it can project as a filling defect from the lateral aspect of the uterus if it is attached to the lateral wall. A sessile myoma, located in the myometrium and the endometrium, projects as a more subtle defect (Figure 6.9). The diagnosis of an intramural myoma that causes

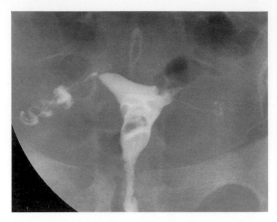

Figure 6.8 Hysterosalpingogram showing a polyp.

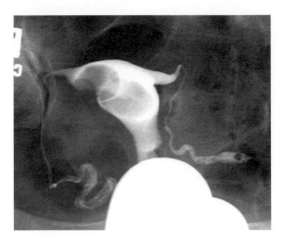

Figure 6.9 Hysterosalpingogram showing a sessile myoma.

deviation of the endometrial cavity is more difficult, since normal anatomic variations or suboptimal positioning of the cavity, either anteverted or retroflexed, can have the appearance of deflection of the cavity. Most women with adenomyosis have a normal HSG, but if the endometrium appears to have small localized diverticula, it is almost always caused by adenomyosis (Figure 6.10). HSG can also identify other uterine anomalies including congenital anomalies or uterine synechia (Figure 6.10).

Assessment of the fallopian tubes can help in surgical planning for a woman with abnormal bleeding, especially for women who desire future pregnancy, and in the case of hematosalpinx, can aid in establishing the diagnosis of abnormal

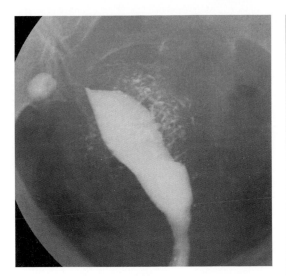

Figure 6.10 Hysterosalpingogram showing adenomyosis.

uterine bleeding. For example, if an infertile woman with abnormal uterine bleeding has bilateral hydrosalpinges, uterine distortion from fibroids, and is not willing to consider IVF, hysterectomy may be a reasonable option.

Another example is the infertile woman who is planning myomectomy: it is better to identify if she has hydrosalpinges before surgery than to be surprised by this finding during operation. If the presence of hydrosalpinges is not identified, the surgeon is left with the following difficult decisions: (1) to perform salpingectomies to optimize future IVF outcomes; (2) to repair the tubes intraoperatively, understanding that a hydrosalpinx may recur after surgical opening and require later removal; or (3) to leave the hydrosalpinges untreated and discuss the findings with the patient postoperatively, knowing that subsequent surgery will be required. Clearly, none of these three choices is optimal for the woman without her prior knowledge and consent, and choosing "incorrectly" during surgery can expose the provider to legal risk.

Finally, if conservative surgery is performed on a woman with infertility, and a subsequent HSG shows proximal tubal occlusion, it would be beneficial to know if the tubes were occluded prior to surgery so the patient can have optimal informed consent before surgery.

> ### ✋ CAUTION
>
> Contraindications for performing hysterosalpingography (HSG) are similar to contraindications to saline infusion sonohysterography. Since HSG involves radiographs, the test should never be done during pregnancy or if pregnancy is suspected. Ideally, HSG should be performed in the follicular phase, after bleeding has stopped and before ovulation. For a patient with excessive irregular bleeding, it is helpful to obtain a progesterone level and a pregnancy test the day of or day before the HSG. A level less than 2 ng/mL indicates that ovulation has not yet occurred. The HSG can be done any time except during withdrawal bleeding for a woman using hormonal contraception. The cervix is prepared with betadine or another antimicrobial solution before placement of the catheter. Antibiotic prophylaxis is not routinely recommended, but if a hydrosalpinx is identified, a broad-spectrum antibiotic such as doxycycline 100 mg twice daily should be prescribed for 10 days to reduce the risk of pelvic infection. HSG should never be performed in a patient with an active pelvic infection or a woman with an allergy to intravenous iodine contrast.

Magnetic resonance imaging

MRI provides the greatest sensitivity for assessing uterine myometrial anatomic abnormalities but should not be ordered unless the test results will alter management. MRI with gadolinium contrast provides the most accurate information about the size, number, and location of uterine fibroids (Figure 6.11). We use MRI to determine appropriate candidates for laparoscopic myomectomy in women with symptomatic fibroids who wish to retain fertility. This technique is often preferred by interventional radiologists to determine appropriate candidates for uterine artery embolization. Furthermore, MRI is required for treatment of fibroids by MRI-guided focused ultrasound surgery.

MRI is more sensitive than ultrasound at differentiating fibroids and adenomyosis (Figure 6.12). Although this differentiation is not impor-

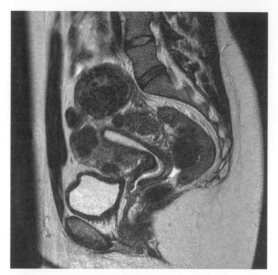

Figure 6.11 Magnetic resonance imaging demonstrating uterine fibroids.

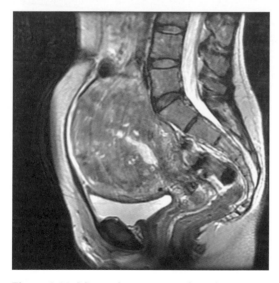

Figure 6.12 Magnetic resonance imaging demonstrating adenomyosis.

tant if hysterectomy is planned, it is a very important factor in determining conservative surgical management for a woman who desires future fertility, since resection and repair of a uterine segment with diffuse adenomyosis is difficult. Most reproductive surgeons avoid resection of adenomyosis because of the unsatisfactory result. Therefore, if MRI findings of adenomyosis would alter management, the higher cost of the test can be justified. MRI can also provide an optimal image of uterine anomalies, can help direct surgery, and is a sensitive imaging test for arteriovenous malformation.

Hysteroscopy

Hysteroscopy can be combined as a diagnostic and therapeutic tool, and some providers find office hysteroscopy more helpful than SIS or HSG in establishing a diagnosis in a woman with abnormal uterine bleeding. As with SIS and HSG, office hysteroscopy should only be performed in the follicular phase, after cessation of menses and before ovulation. It is important to use a thin hysteroscope to avoid the need to dilate the cervix and to reduce cramping, and flexible hysteroscopy is preferred. Gas is used to distend the cavity. The procedure is usually well tolerated, but pretreatment with ibuprofen improves patient comfort. Office hysteroscopy is an appropriate method to assess polyps in the uterus or cervix, submucous or sessile fibroids, or endometrial inflammation or hypertrophy. A drawback of office hysteroscopy is the expense and limited availability of the hysteroscopy system, as well as the possible need to perform operative hysteroscopy at a later time if a treatable abnormality is identified.

Ancillary testing

Additional testing may markedly affect management options for a woman who desires future fertility, even though it seems unrelated to the diagnosis and treatment of abnormal uterine bleeding. A semen analysis and ovarian reserve testing should be considered in addition to ultrasound and HSG for a woman with abnormal bleeding and infertility. Ovarian reserve testing can be done by obtaining follicle-stimulating hormone (FSH) and estradiol between cycle days 1 and 5, determining the number of follicles 2–9 mm in size in each ovary to assess the antral follicle count, or measuring antimüllerian hormone level. Variations have been reported from one center to another, but a basal FSH level higher than 15 mIU/mL, basal estradiol greater than 70 pg/mL, basal antral follicle count below 10, or antimüllerian hormone level below 1.0 ng/mL has been associated with diminished ovarian reserve and reduced prognosis with fertility treatments.

In order to see how these tests alter decisions, consider a 42-year-old infertile woman with five large fibroids and abnormal uterine bleeding with an elevated FSH level; her husband's semen analysis shows azoospermia (no sperm). This patient might prefer hysterectomy instead of myomectomy, since the prognosis for fertility after conservative surgery is remote. However, if the semen analysis and ovarian reserve testing is normal, she may choose myomectomy to alleviate symptoms and preserve fertility potential.

Conclusions

The evaluation and treatment of abnormal uterine bleeding due to anatomic abnormalities begins with confirmation of ovulation and concurrent identification of the abnormality. Laboratory tests and imaging studies are used to confirm the diagnosis. Polyps, fibroids, or adenomyosis is usually the cause mechanical abnormal bleeding.

Selected bibliography

Aliyu MH, Aliyu SH, Salihu HM. Female genital tuberculosis: a global review. Int J Fertil Womens Med 2004;49:123–36.

Clark TJ. Outpatient hysteroscopy and ultrasonography in the management of endometrial disease. Cur Opin Obstet Gynecol 2004;16:305–11.

de Kroon CD, de Bock GH, Dieben SW, Jansen FW. Saline contrast hysterosonography in abnormal uterine bleeding: a systematic review and meta-analysis. BJOG 2003;110:938–47.

Ducatman BS. Pathologic diagnosis of the abnormally bleeding patient. Clin Obstet Gynecol 2005;48:274–83.

ESHRE Capri Workshop Group, Collins J, Crosignani PG. Endometrial bleeding. Hum Reprod Update 2007;13:421–31.

Farquhar C, Brown J. Oral contraceptive pill for heavy menstrual bleeding. Cochrane Database Syst Rev 2009, Issue 4. Art. No.: CD000154.

Hatasaka H. The evaluation of abnormal uterine bleeding. Clin Obstet Gynecol 2005;48:258–73.

Lasmar RB, Dias R, Barrozo PR, Oliveira MA, Coutinho Eda S, da Rosa DB. Prevalence of hysteroscopic findings and histologic diagnoses in patients with abnormal uterine bleeding. Fertil Steril 2008;89:1803–7.

Levgur M. Diagnosis of adenomyosis: a review. J Reprod Med 2007;52:177–93.

Nathani F, Clark TJ. Uterine polypectomy in the management of abnormal uterine bleeding: a systematic review. J Minimally Invasive Gynecol 2006;13:260–8.

Pallone SR, Bergus GR. Fertility awareness-based methods: another option for family planning. J Am Board Family Med 2009;22:147–57.

Practice Committee of American Society for Reproductive Medicine in collaboration with Society for Reproductive Endocrinology and Infertility. Optimizing natural fertility. Fertil Steril 2008;90:S1–6.

Valentin L. Imaging in gynecology. Best Practice Res Clin Obstet Gynaecol 2006;20:881–906.

van Dongen H, de Kroon CD, Jacobi CE, Trimbos JB, Jansen FW. Diagnostic hysteroscopy in abnormal uterine bleeding: a systematic review and meta-analysis. BJOG 2007;114:664–75.

Van Voorhis B. A 41-year-old woman with menorrhagia, anemia, and fibroids: review of treatment of uterine fibroids. JAMA 2009;301:82–93.

7

Abnormal Uterine Bleeding due to Anatomic Causes: Treatment

Bradley S. Hurst

Carolinas Medical Center, Charlotte, North Carolina, USA

The patient hemodynamically unstable due to anatomic abnormality

Stabilization and control of hemorrhage are the first two steps for a woman with abnormal uterine bleeding due to an anatomic abnormality. The patient should be observed in a monitored setting, one or two large-bore intravenous lines placed, and a large fluid bolus, 500–1000 mL initially, given with physiologic crystalloids such as lactated Ringer's solution or normal saline, 500–1000 mL initially and then 125–150 mL per hour continuously. A complete blood count, pregnancy test, and blood type and crossmatch are immediately obtained. If blood is needed, the use of matched blood is preferable over type O negative blood, unless immediate transfusion is required.

Tranexamic acid reduces bleeding by approximately 50% and should be administered to a woman with life-threatening hemorrhage unless contraindicated. Tranexamic acid is an antifibrinolytic agent that inhibits the activation of plasminogen to plasmin and is approved by the Food and Drug Administration for treatment of menorrhagia. The approved dose of tranexamic acid (Lysteda) is two 650 mg pills (1300 mg) three times daily for up to 5 days. The most common side effects include headache, sinus and nasal symptoms, back pain, abdominal pain, muscle and joint pain, muscle cramps, anemia, and fatigue.

> ✋ **CAUTION**
>
> Concurrent use of tranexamic acid and hormonal contraceptives may increase the risk of blood clots, stroke, or heart attack. Women using hormonal contraception should use tranexamic acid only if the benefit outweighs the potential risks.

As hemodynamic stability is restored, attention turns to controlling the bleeding. Unlike the anovulatory patient who is usually stabilized with hormonal management, high-dose estrogen or oral contraceptives are less effective with mechanical causes. Even if they appear to be successful initially, hormonal treatment may contribute to a severe delayed bleeding episode. Mechanical methods are more appropriate to directly tamponade or coagulate the bleeding vessels.

Observation is the simplest measure to control bleeding for a woman with a polyp or fibroid. In most cases, the heaviest bleeding will lessen after 6–12 hours as the vessels clot. If observation is not appropriate due to the severity of the bleeding, the woman with an anatomic abnor-

Disorders of Menstruation, 1st edition. Edited by Paul B. Marshburn and Bradley S. Hurst.
© 2011 Blackwell Publishing Ltd.

mality will probably achieve greater control with mechanical measures. A balloon catheter (such as a Foley urinary catheter with a 10 mL balloon) placed into the uterus and inflated tamponades the bleeding vessels. Placement is simple and will control the bleeding if the site of hemorrhage corresponds with the site of the inflated balloon, so use of a 10 mL balloon is more effective than a 3 mL balloon. If this method is successful, the balloon is removed after 24–72 hours. The catheter can be replaced if hemorrhage resumes.

If hemorrhage continues in spite of these measures, it can be diagnostic and therapeutic to perform a hysteroscopy. A high-flow saline system with suction overflow should be used for distention to flush the blood and allow adequate visualization. If identified, bleeding vessels can be coagulated with a bipolar wire or loop electrode to control the bleeding. If bleeding is diffuse and is occurring throughout the endometrium, circumferential endometrial curettage may be helpful to control the bleeding. If bleeding slows but still occurs at a higher than ideal rate, a balloon catheter can be inflated in the cavity to reduce blood flow. A triangular intrauterine balloon catheter may more completely tamponade bleeding and minimize focal compression than a spherical balloon. There have been anecdotal reports of intrauterine adhesions from presumed ischemia after prolonged use of an inflated Foley catheter balloon.

It is unusual for these measures to fail, and if bleeding continues further, hematologic studies are needed to evaluate for coagulopathy. These include repeat complete blood count, prothrombin time/partial thromboplastin time, and fibrinogen split products; abnormalities should be addressed as well. Other measures may be considered, depending on the patient's desire for fertility. If she wishes to preserve fertility, uterine artery embolization (UAE) therapy will reduce the uterine bleeding acutely. If future fertility is not desired and endometrial carcinoma is excluded, endometrial ablation will acutely control the bleeding. If other measures fail, hysterectomy may be required. However, before hysterectomy, all attempts must be made to ensure that the patient is hemodynamically stable and the coagulopathy corrected.

Following stabilization, care is provided to evaluate the problem and provide the most appropriate treatment. This depends on the underlying etiology as determined by the evaluation described in this chapter, the woman's desire for future fertility, her age and general health, and her desire for uterine preservation.

Polyps

Polyps arise from the endometrium or the endocervix, and although there are no known causative factors, polyps respond grow in response to estrogen and progesterone exposure. Polyps are composed of fibrous stromal tissue, vessels, and endometrial epithelial glands. Approximately 10% of women develop polyps, with a higher incidence in obese women. Polyps are present in approximately 25% of women with abnormal uterine bleeding. Symptoms attributed to an endometrial polyp include menorrhagia, dysmenorrhea, clotting with menses, and intermenstrual bleeding, although many women are asymptomatic. Hysteroscopic polypectomy appears to be beneficial in women with infertility.

Endometrial polyps can be identified by ultrasonography, saline infusion sonography, or hysterosalpingography (Figure 7.1). When a polypoid mass is identified, the differential diagnosis in a reproductive-aged woman is limited to a polyp or submucous myoma. Polyps may be solitary or multiple. The incidence of adenocarcinoma in a suspected polyp is approximately 1 in 1000. Once a polyp has been identified in a symptomatic woman, treatment should be offered with the goals of a cost-effective approach, high rate of success, and minimal risk.

Historically, cervical dilatation and endometrial and cervical curettage (D&C) have been the initial treatment for a woman with suspected polyps, but since polyps can be completely missed by D&C, hysteroscopic polypectomy is now the standard of care. Hysteroscopy allows direct visualization and confirmation of removal, and symptoms should cease (Figure 7.2).

Hysteroscopy is performed in the follicular phase of the menstrual cycle, ideally after menstrual bleeding stops and before ovulation. Hysteroscopy can be performed at any time except during withdrawal bleeding for a woman

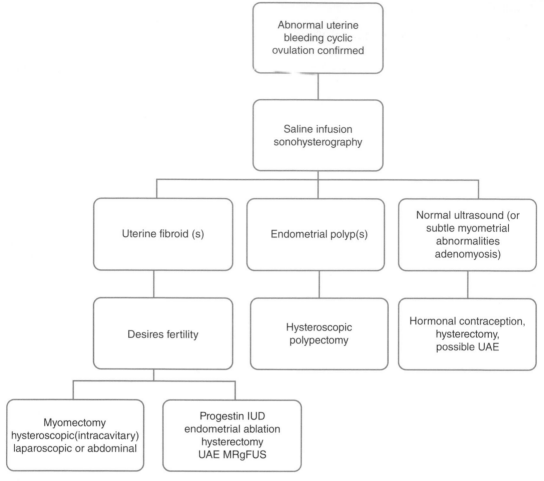

Figure 7.1 Management of abnormal uterine bleeding due to anatomic causes. See text for abbreviations.

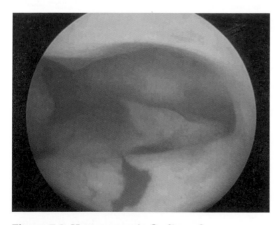

Figure 7.2 Hysteroscopic finding of an endometrial polyp (see Plate 7.2).

using hormonal contraception. If the polyp is large, or if it is unclear whether the intracavitary mass is a polyp or a fibroid, visualization is improved by pretreatment with a gonadotropin-releasing hormone (GnRH) agonist such as leuprolide 3.75 mg administered on day 21 in the cycle before surgery. After the GnRH agonist has been given and once the next menstrual cycle starts, estradiol levels remain low and the endometrium stays thin, allowing optimal visualization during the surgery. Alternatively, the endometrium becomes thin after 2–3 months of hormonal contraception. GnRH agonist therapy or hormonal contraception eventually reduces bleeding, allowing a severely anemic patient to recover in preparation for surgery.

Placement of a tablet of misoprostol 400 µg into the vagina the night before surgery makes cervical dilatation safer and easier. Misoprostol is a prostaglandin, and side effects may include cramping, spotting, loose stools, or nausea, but it is usually tolerated well by patients preparing for hysteroscopy. Prophylactic antibiotics are not recommended.

Hysteroscopic polypectomy is performed in the operating room under general anesthesia or sedation. The bladder is emptied, and a speculum is placed into the vagina. An examination is helpful to determine the size and position of the uterus. A tenaculum is placed on the anterior cervix to straighten the cervical canal, and the cervix is progressively dilated to accommodate the hysteroscope. The hysteroscope is placed into the uterus, and in most cases saline is used to distend the endometrial cavity. A flow meter records inflow pressure, total fluid inflow, and return, in order to avoid causing a large fluid deficit (over 1000 mL), which could cause dangerous electrolyte problems. The major anatomic landmarks should be identified, including both tubal ostia, the uterine body, and the cervix. The polyp can be removed under direct visualization with hysteroscopic scissors, grasping forceps, or a resectoscopic loop, with or without electrical energy. The polyp or polyp fragments should be recovered and sent for histologic examination to confirm the diagnosis and exclude hyperplasia or carcinoma.

If equipment or visualization is not adequate to directly remove the polyp by hysteroscopy, an endometrial curettage can be performed. Once the polypoid mass has been removed, the hysteroscope can be placed back into the uterus to confirm satisfactory polypectomy. Visualization is limited and bleeding can occur following curettage, so direct removal under hysteroscopic visualization is preferred.

Postoperatively, the patient may experience cramping for 1–2 days, and ibuprofen is effective in most cases. Unlimited activities may resume the day after hysteroscopy, but the patient should avoid intercourse, douching, and tampons until bleeding has stopped in order to prevent the risk of ascending infection. Attempts to conceive can begin in the cycle following hysteroscopic polypectomy.

A woman with abnormal uterine bleeding due to an endometrial polyp may consider endometrial ablation after she has completed childbearing, as long as endometrial adenocarcinoma has been excluded by biopsy. Endometrial ablation is performed in a number of techniques, but hysteroscopic polypectomy may be done immediately before ablation since there is a small possibility of focal endometrial cancer in a polyp. Hysteroscopic rollerball ablation has been mostly replaced by ablation devices such as balloon ablation or ablation with a bipolar ablation.

Approximately 90% of women experience a reduction in menstrual bleeding, and some women develop amenorrhea. Pregnancy is unlikely following endometrial ablation, so this procedure should not be considered if future fertility is desired. However, ablation is not a contraceptive method, so contraception is needed for the premenopausal sexually active woman. A return to normal or lighter bleeding normally follows ablation. More invasive measures such as hysterectomy are not appropriate for the management of a simple benign endometrial polyp, unless also used for other indications.

It is possible that hormonal contraception or use of a progestin intrauterine device (IUD) can reduce menorrhagia and dysmenorrhea in a woman with a uterine polyp. While these may be temporizing measures, neither results in resolution of the underlying problem: the polyp. In most circumstances, surgical removal is needed for reproductive-aged women with abnormal uterine bleeding attributed to a polyp.

Fibroids

The uterine fibroid deforms the surrounding tissues as it grows. The fibroid is surrounded by a dense vascular capsule, and small vessels penetrate into the mass. In general, larger tumors have greater vascularity. A fibroid that develops within the myometrium is considered an "intramural" myoma. If the fibroid causes distortion of the endometrium, it is a submucous myoma, and if the fibroid distorts the serosa, it is termed a subserosal myoma. The term "sessile" refers to a fibroid that is located in the myometrium but also distorts the endometrium. A pedunculated fibroid develops primarily outside the uterus, sometimes on a stalk connected to the uterus. Abnormal bleeding is attributed to fibroids that directly distort the endometrium, to submucous and sessile myomas, or to intramural myomas that indirectly enlarge the endometrial cavity, but not to most intramural, subserosal, or pedunculated myomas. For this discussion, the terms "fibroid," "myoma," and "leiomyoma" are used interchangeably.

The incidence of uterine fibroids peaks during the fourth decade because estrogen and progesterone stimulate their growth. There is a clear predisposition to fibroids in women of African descent, and fibroids are more numerous and larger in this group. However, fibroids are common in all racial groups. Ultrasound studies have shown that fibroids exist in as many as 89% of African-American women and 70% of Caucasian women. There is great interest in identifying dietary and environmental factors for fibroids, but no clear association has been found.

Most women with fibroids are asymptomatic, although many with abnormal uterine bleeding due to anatomic causes have uterine fibroids, and fibroids are the leading indication for hysterectomy. Symptoms associated with fibroids related to endometrial distortion include menorrhagia, dysmenorrhea, menstrual clotting, and intermenstrual bleeding. When bleeding is severe, anemia may occur. A uterus that is enlarged from fibroids may cause bulk symptoms such as abdominal pressure, bloating, or distention. If a myoma is pressing against the bladder, urinary frequency, urgency, or nocturia may occur. If there is pressure against the rectum, constipation, diarrhea, or alternating symptoms can occur. Fibroids may be painful in several circumstances, and infarction of a myoma can lead to intense acute pain. If a fibroid is located in the posterior cul-de-sac, it can cause dyspareunia. Some women experience chronic pain, intermittent pain, or cyclic pain associated with fibroids.

Uterine fibroids can cause infertility or poor reproductive outcomes. Infertility is usually attributed to submucous or sessile myomas that directly distort the endometrial cavity. Additionally, there are increasing data suggesting that intramural fibroids reduce fertility, especially when they are 4 cm or larger in size. Myomectomy appears to restore fertility. Women who have uterine fibroids have a significantly higher risk of delivering a baby with low birth weight, placental abruption, breech presentation, and premature rupture of membranes. The incidence of cesarean section is increased, and there is a higher risk of requiring a maternal blood transfusion after delivery because of postpartum hemorrhage.

Treatment considerations

The provider must consider a number of factors in order to determine the most appropriate treatment for uterine myomas, but a general principle is to select the most cost-effective, least invasive approach with the lowest risk that also provides the greatest efficacy and shortest recovery (see Figure 7.1 above). Unfortunately, in many cases no one procedure meets all of these objectives.

In most circumstances, a pragmatic approach is to consider treatment based on symptoms, physical findings, and patient desires. For example, hysterectomy is not appropriate for a woman who desires future fertility or who strongly wishes to preserve her uterus, but it might be an excellent choice for a woman who has multiple symptoms associated with fibroids and prefers a permanent resolution. The size, number, and location of fibroids need to be considered when treatment is planned, and risks and benefits of each option should be assessed individually; there is no "one size fits all" solution. Importantly, local resources must be taken into account, and some treatments are not available in all regions. Finally, the skill, training, and experience of the surgeon may limit some treatment options.

Treatment options for uterine fibroids and abnormal uterine bleeding

Expectant management is appropriate for women who have minor, tolerable symptoms. Although fibroids usually grow and symptoms worsen over a period of time, observation can be a reasonable choice when the patient is uncertain about her treatment decision. As symptoms progress, the fear of surgery may become less than the severity of the symptoms and help the patient choose the best treatment option.

Observation may also be appropriate for a woman who is clearly close to menopause, since fibroids are expected to shrink and become less symptomatic in the postmenopausal years. If a woman chooses observation, it is reasonable to perform clinical updates of fibroid-related symptoms and physical and pelvic examination at approximately 6-month intervals if fibroids are enlarging and 12-month intervals if the size and symptoms appear stable. An ultrasound at these intervals may help by providing objective documentation of growth. Observation is not appropriate for a woman if cancer is suspected.

Progestin intrauterine device

The IUD with levonorgestrel, a progestin, reduces menorrhagia and dysmenorrhea in some women with uterine fibroids by causing decidualization and eventual atrophy of the endometrium. This approach is likely to be effective in cases when the uterine cavity has a relatively normal size and shape, and less effective when as the distortion of the cavity is extensive. Although the progestin IUD does not typically cause a reduction in the size or number of fibroids, it is a temporizing measure and is only effective while the IUD is in place. The IUD will have no benefit for bulk symptoms caused by intramural or subserosal myomas. Extra caution is needed during placement of an IUD in a woman with uterine fibroids, since the cervical canal or uterus may be distorted and more prone to perforation while inserting the IUD. The progestin IUD (levonorgestrel intrauterine system) can produce considerable relief in women with uterine enlargement, menorrhagia, and dysmenorrhea secondary to adenomyosis with or without coexistent fibroids.

Other types of hormonal contraception are less effective than the progestin IUD for abnormal uterine bleeding due to uterine fibroids. Nevertheless, it is not unreasonable to attempt a trial of hormonal contraception as long as the patient has no contraindications. Oral contraceptives, transdermal contraceptives, the vaginal contraceptive ring, or depot injectable contraceptives can cause modest relief in some patients.

Gonadotropin-releasing hormone agonists

GnRH agonists are useful in several circumstances for a woman with abnormal uterine bleeding due to fibroids: reducing bleeding so the patient can recover from anemia while preparing for surgery, endometrial preparation to thin the endometrium before hysteroscopic myomectomy, and as a temporizing measure to reduce symptoms in a woman before menopause. Some surgeons prescribe GnRH agonists to reduce uterine volume and enable consideration of vaginal or laparoscopic hysterectomy.

GnRH agonists suppress pituitary secretion of follicle-stimulating hormone and luteinizing hormone and induce a hypoestrogenic state. Fibroids shrink by approximately 50% during treatment, but this holds no long-term benefit because fibroids return to their pretreatment size within 3 months after stopping treatment. Temporary ovarian suppression does stop ovulation and menstrual bleeding, and although "breakthrough bleeding" can occur, bleeding tends to be reduced or stopped during GnRH agonist therapy in most women with uterine fibroids. Allowing recovery of menorrhagia-related anemia improves safety during surgery, and initiating surgery with higher hemoglobin levels reduces the need for transfusion as a result of intraoperative or postoperative bleeding. GnRH agonists have been approved by the U.S. Food and Drug Administration for this indication.

Preoperative use of GnRH agonists has some drawbacks, and they therefore should not be used indiscriminately. Treatment is expensive and this limits use of these drugs only when the benefit is not clearly defined. Furthermore, the hypoestrogenic state caused by treatment results in menopausal vasomotor symptoms and rapid bone loss that can lead to osteopenia or osteoporosis. These side effects prevent long-term use, with the possible exception being a woman who is clearly close to menopause when fibroids will begin to shrink and fibroid-related symptoms will resolve. GnRH agonist pretreatment is helpful to cause endometrial atrophy and improve visualization for hysteroscopic myomectomy, but has sometimes been shown to increase the difficulty of fibroid enucleation, and may increase the risk of recurrence after myomectomy.

Promising temporizing measures

Although there is no medical treatment that "cures" fibroids, several temporizing measures hold promise. Progesterone antagonists have been shown to reduce menorrhagia related to fibroids, and reduce fibroid volume in clinical studies. These drugs are well tolerated, although there are few data exploring long-term safety. Unfortunately, these agents can also cause pregnancy disruption and endometrial hyperplasia, so clinical applications have slowed. Aromatase inhibitors hinder the conversion of androgens to estrogens, and preliminary studies show promising short-term results. Unfortunately, no medical therapy has been evaluated for long-term symptomatic control, and rapid regrowth of fibroids is expected after cessation of any hormonal intervention.

Hysteroscopic myomectomy

Hysteroscopic myomectomy should be considered as the primary approach for a woman with abnormal uterine bleeding attributed to a submucous myoma. Hysteroscopic myomectomy has a tremendous advantage in that it is a safe, simple, cost-effective approach with rapid recovery. In a woman with bulk symptoms, it can be combined with laparoscopic or open myomectomy when fertility or uterine preservation is desired. Even in a woman who has no desire for future fertility, the advantages of hysteroscopic myomectomy compare favorably to those of hysterectomy, the only permanent treatment for fibroids. When used for the post-childbearing woman, hysteroscopic myomectomy can be performed in conjunction with endometrial ablation to improve the long-term effectiveness of the procedure.

The practitioner should perform hysteroscopic myomectomy when the endometrium is thin to achieve optimal visualization. This can be accomplished by performing the hysteroscopy in the follicular phase of the cycle, but it may be difficult to schedule at the ideal time in the cycle since menstrual bleeding can obscure visualization, and bleeding is typically heavier and longer in a woman with a submucous myoma. In order to overcome these problems, it is beneficial to prepare the endometrium hormonally with

GnRH agonists and oral contraceptives. Danazol, an androgen analog, is also used effectively for this purpose, but androgenic side effects preclude its widespread use.

GnRH agonists may cause initial pituitary stimulation, but this is overcome by administering a 1-month dose of the drug in the midluteal phase. In the United States, leuprolide acetate 3.75 mg is most commonly used GnRH agonist. Once menses occur, the endometrium remains thin at least for 28 days from administration, so surgery can be scheduled for any time within this window. Repeat doses are not needed. Alternatively, oral contraceptives are effective at preparing the endometrium and much less expensive than GnRH agonists, but the endometrial thins more slowly and presurgical treatment for 2–3 months may be required. This delay is problematic in cases with heavy breakthrough bleeding.

Hysteroscopic myomectomy techniques are similar to those used for polypectomy, with a few important exceptions. Hysteroscopic myomectomy is accomplished most efficiently with a loop resectoscope (Figure 7.3). Modern hysteroscopic systems monitor inflow pressure and fluid deficit to prevent complications that arise from excessive fluid absorption and electrolyte disturbances. Pressure should be kept as low as possible to provide distension of the cavity but avoid intravasation of fluids; a pressure of approximately 80 mmHg is usually adequate. The hysteroscopic

surgery should be stopped if the deficit becomes too great, usually approximately 1000 mL. Because of this limitation, it might be necessary to remove a large fibroid in two separate procedures. Additionally, the myoma should only be resected to the level of the endometrium, and not into the myometrium, in order to avoid perforation of the uterus and potential damage to adjacent organs. This is not a problem for a submucous myoma, but care is needed while resecting a sessile myoma.

☆ TIPS & TRICKS

During hysteroscopic myomectomy, the resectoscope loop is placed distal to the fibroid, and then the loop is activated and slowly retracted towards the hysteroscope. The loop should never be advanced while activated as this can cause uterine perforation. An experienced surgeon will remove as many strips of the myoma as possible until the fragments obscure visualization. Once visualization is compromised, the fragments can be removed with polyp forceps or a gentle circular sweep of the cavity with a large curette. The process is repeated until the submucous fibroid is completely resected, or until a sessile myoma is resected to the level of the endometrium. After a few minutes, the residual sessile myoma may herniate into the cavity as the myometrium contracts, and additional tissue can be removed. If any myoma remains, one of three outcomes may occur: it may become covered by the endometrium, migrate further into the myometrium and become asymptomatic, or herniate further into the cavity and later require an additional resectoscopic procedure.

Bleeding is usually light after hysteroscopic myomectomy, but if heavy bleeding occurs a balloon catheter can be placed into the uterus and inflated, which usually tamponades the bleeding site and allows formation of a blood clot. The catheter should be removed within a few days to limit the risk of uterine adhesions from pressure necrosis from an overinflated balloon.

The endometrium heals approximately 6 weeks after hysteroscopic myomectomy, and

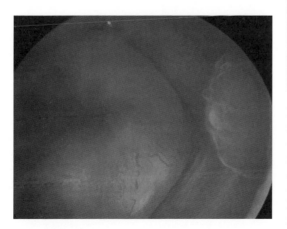

Figure 7.3 Hysteroscopic myomectomy (see Plate 7.3).

pregnancy should be postponed until healing is complete. The first period after this procedure may be heavier than subsequent periods since the cavity is still healing

Endometrial ablation

Endometrial ablation by a balloon, mesh, or hysteroscopic rollerball can be performed after completion of hysteroscopic myomectomy for women who are beyond the childbearing years. The bipolar mesh device may also be used as primary treatment when the uterine cavity measures 10 cm or less. By comparison, a hysteroscopic rollerball ablation can be performed regardless of the size or shape of the cavity since it is performed under direct observation.

Myomectomy

Myomectomy is an appropriate treatment for symptomatic fibroids if fertility or uterine preservation is desired and when more conservative measures such as hysteroscopic myomectomy will not alleviate symptoms. Large, multiple fibroids that cause bulk symptoms may be removed, as may submucous and sessile myomas. Preoperative ultrasound or magnetic resonance imaging (MRI) to determine the size, number, and location of uterine fibroids provide invaluable information to help plan the surgery. These imaging modalities can also exclude adenomyosis, which can be difficult to treat surgically.

Myomectomy may be performed as an open procedure, at the time of laparotomy, or as a laparoscopic procedure. In all cases, removal of all submucous or sessile myomas is crucial to accomplish the greatest relief for the woman with abnormal uterine bleeding. Hysteroscopic resection might be a useful aid in some circumstances. The approach is chosen based on the size, number, and location of the fibroids, and the skill of the surgeon.

Abdominal myomectomy

The first cases of abdominal myomectomy were published in 1845 by the brothers Washington and John Atlee in the *American Journal of Medical Science*. Washington Atlee won the American Medical Association prize paper for their experience with 14 myomectomies, even though five women died from surgical complications!

By the beginning of the twentieth century, the abdominal myomectomy mortality rate was still approximately 40%, and the procedure was therefore reserved for the most serious cases. This changed rapidly in the 1920s, when Victor Bonney and others reported outstanding outcomes with their techniques. Although the procedure is now safer because of the improvements in anesthesia, antiseptic agents, and new techniques and instruments, surprisingly little change has occurred in methodology since that time.

Abdominal myomectomy is performed through an incision that allows adequate exposure to complete the task of removing all possible fibroids and repairing the uterus. Most surgeons prefer a Pfannenstiel incision. Selective myomectomy can be done through a smaller incision initially to provide more exposure. A Maylard rectus muscle cutting entry can provide greater exposure through a transverse incision when the uterus is massively enlarged, although some surgeons still prefer the exposure gained from a midline laparotomy for extreme cases.

Hemostatic measures should be incorporated into all myomectomy procedures. We prefer injecting the myoma pseudocapsule with a dilute solution of vasopressin, with 10 U diluted by 10 mL saline. Injection with 1–3 mL of this solution is usually sufficient to constrict the myoma vasculature and limit bleeding. Other techniques utilized include a local anesthetic such as lidocaine with epinephrine (adrenaline), or use of a tourniquet to mechanically constrict the uterine vasculature. It is important to monitor blood pressure while using these agents, since transient hypertension can occur with intravascular injections.

★ TIPS & TRICKS

Uterine incisions should be planned to remove the largest number of fibroids through the fewest incisions. The uterine incision is carried down to the fibroid, and because the density of the fibroid is different from that of the normal myometrium, the myoma pseudocapsule is easily defined. The myoma is then separated from the myometrium by electrocautery dissection, blunt dissection, or sharp dissection, with great care taken at the base of each fibroid to avoid damage to the endometrium. Once a fibroid has been removed, adjacent fibroids can be pushed into the incision and dissected through the myometrium to avoid further disrupting the serosa or enlarging the incision if possible. Great care must be taken when removing fibroids near the fallopian tubes to minimize the risk of tubal damage, and when dissecting fibroids in the broad ligament area to avoid harming these vessels or the ureter.

A systematic approach is optimal as it is possible to remove many fibroids through a single incision. The incision is repaired in multiple layers including an endometrial closure, if the endometrium was entered during the myomectomy, involving a deep myometrial layer, a superficial myometrial layer, and a serosal layer. The final serosal layer should be closed with minimal tension to limit the risk of incision separation. Once the incision has been closed, more incisions can be made to remove additional fibroids, followed by repair. This process is repeated until all visible and palpable fibroids have been removed.

Adhesion barriers should be used to minimize the risk of postmyomectomy adhesions. Randomized clinical trials have shown that adhesions form in over 90% of fundal and posterior myomectomy incisions, and oxidized regenerated cellulose (Interceed; Johnson & Johnson, New Brunswick, NJ, USA), hyaluronic acid (Seprafilm; Genzyme, Cambridge, MA, USA), and Preclude (WL Gore, Flagstaff, AZ, USA) have been shown to reduce adhesions after myomectomy. Pregnancy should be avoided for approximately 3 months while the uterus heals.

Women with multiple fibroids are more likely to have recurrent fibroids and to require subsequent surgery compared to women who have one or two myomas. Of all women who undergo myomectomy, approximately 60% will have recurrent fibroids, and approximately 15–25% will require subsequent intervention. Although the risk of incision separation during labor is less than 1% for an uncomplicated myomectomy, most surgeons in the United States recommend delivery by cesarean section, since uterine rupture during labor can have catastrophic consequences for the mother and the fetus.

Laparoscopic myomectomy

Laparoscopic myomectomy was first described by Semm in the 1970s. Early instruments were fairly crude, and few surgeons took on the challenge of laparoscopic myomectomy until the 1990s, when rapid improvement in instruments and techniques allowed endoscopic surgeons to use acceptable techniques for removing fibroids and repairing the myomectomy incisions.

Compared to the open approach, laparoscopic myomectomy provides several advantages in randomized clinical trials, including less pain, less postoperative fever, shorter hospitalization, a shorter recovery interval, and, in some studies, reduced blood loss. The surgical time, subsequent pregnancy rates, and fibroid recurrence rates are similar when performed by skilled surgeons. Postoperative patient satisfaction also appears similar between the two approaches.

Laparoscopic myomectomy is performed at some centers with robotic surgery, but can also be performed by an experienced laparoscopic surgical team. Key points for performing laparoscopic myomectomy include proper patient selection, optimal trocar port placement to provide adequate exposure, traction, and countertraction during the procedure, and adequate tools to facilitate the procedure. Preoperative MRI scanning with gadolinium contrast provides the greatest information about the size, number, and location of fibroids (Figure 7.4). There is a limit to the number and size of fibroids that can be removed during laparoscopic myomectomy; therefore abdominal myomectomy can be a more prudent approach when fibroids are massive (greater than 10–14 cm) or multiple (more than five), unless the surgical team has extensive experience with complex laparoscopic myomectomy cases.

⚠ CAUTION

Small sessile myomas present a particularly difficult problem for laparoscopic myomectomy, since these masses may not be detected during laparoscopy. If a sessile myoma is present and laparoscopic myomectomy

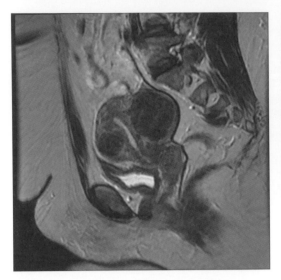

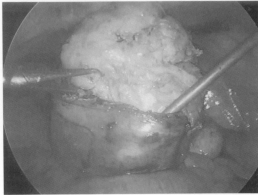

Figure 7.5 Laparoscopic myomectomy initial incision (see Plate 7.5).

Figure 7.4 Magnetic resonance imaging demonstrating uterine fibroids in a patient considering laparoscopic myomectomy.

planned, it might be beneficial to perform an intraoperative vaginal or intra-abdominal ultrasound to determine the location of the myoma, which allows for an appropriate incision site. Additionally, magnetic resonance imaging helps differentiate myomas and adenomyosis. Laparoscopic resection of diffuse adenomyosis is challenging, and repair following excision can be extremely difficult; in addition, there is no proven benefit for resection on subsequent fertility. For that reason, when adenomyosis is identified, it is appropriate to consider medical treatment.

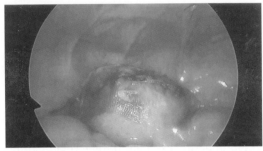

Figure 7.6 Laparoscopic myomectomy placement of an adhesion barrier (see Plate 7.6).

When the uterus is large, the initial incision can be placed at Palmer's point, two to three finger-breadths below the left costal margin near the midclavicular line, after a nasogastric tube has decompressed the stomach. A second incision is placed to the right of the umbilicus and in the right lower quadrant, both lateral to the epigastric vessels. A 12 mm incision is placed in the left lower quadrant, to be used for myoma traction during dissection, assisting suturing, and myoma morcellation. The myoma pseudocapsule is injected with a vasoconstrictive agent such as vasopressin 10 units in 10 mL saline, and the myoma dissected from the pseudocapsule with a hemostatic cutting device, such as a Harmonic Scalpel hook (Ethicon—Johnson & Johnson; Figure 7.5). The fibroid masses are removed with a mechanical morcellator, and an adhesion barrier should be placed over the incision lines to reduce the risk of postoperative adhesions (Figure 7.6).

Once the fibroid has been removed, the uterus is closed in multiple layers, as is performed for open myomectomy. Use of a self-righting needle driver facilitates closure of each layer with a running layer of an absorbable minimally reactive suture, and Lapra-Ty clips (Ethicon—Johnson & Johnson) placed on the sutures saves time by limiting or preventing the need to tie sutures during laparoscopy.

Postoperatively, most women return home on the day of surgery and can resume full activities within 2 weeks of surgery. The first menses may be slightly heavier than expected, due to uterine healing, especially if a sessile myoma has been removed. Pregnancy should be avoided for 3 months to allow for uterine healing. Delivery by cesarean section will reduce the risk of uterine incision separation during labor. Although this risk of dehiscence is small after laparoscopic myomectomy, approximately one case in 100, the consequences can be tragic to the mother and fetus.

Uterine artery embolization

UAE, sometimes referred to as "uterine fibroid embolization," is performed by interventional radiologists by injecting occluding particles such as microspheres or polyvinyl alcohol into the right and left uterine arteries through a femoral arterial approach during fluoroscopy, while the patient is sedated. The particles flow into the uterine vasculature, but since the myoma vessels are large there tends to be selective flow into the myoma vasculature. Infarction due to lack of perfusion eventually causes the fibroid to shrink. The more normal myometrium and endometrium are perfused with collateral vessels, so diffuse uterine infarction does not occur.

UAE was first reported in 1979 for postpartum hemorrhage and hemorrhage following gynecologic surgery. UAE was first described as a treatment for fibroids by Ravina in Paris in 1995, initially as an adjunct to myomectomy and then as primary treatment. When the first cases of UAE were published in the United States by McLucas and colleagues in Los Angeles in 1996, the breakthrough in fibroid therapy was reported in the national news. The procedure is widely available, and more than 10,000 UAE procedures are performed in the United States annually.

Results with UAE are consistent among experienced centers. Uterine volume decreases approximately 50%, and 85–90% of women have a significant improvement in bleeding, pain, and bulk symptoms. Patient satisfaction rates and quality of life scores are high after UAE.

UAE is the most appropriate choice for symptomatic fibroids after childbearing has been completed in women who wish to avoid hyster-

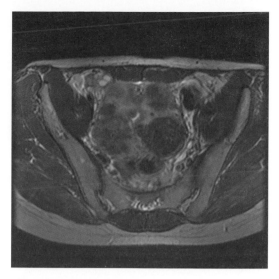

Figure 7.7 Magnetic resonance imaging showing "innumerable fibroids."

ectomy and who are poor surgical candidates. UAE may be the best or only option for women who desire fertility when "innumerable" small fibroids are identified, since it may not be possible to remove all of the potentially problematic myomas and perform a satisfactory repair during myomectomy (Figure 7.7). UAE can also be considered for women who have recurrent fibroids after myomectomy or other conservative treatment. However, women with isolated submucous myomas should be treated by hysteroscopic myomectomy and not UAE, since hysteroscopic surgery provides excellent symptomatic relief, more rapid recovery, and a lower cost than UAE. Women who desire a permanent solution for fibroids should consider hysterectomy, since subsequent treatment is required for persistent or recurrent symptoms in 20–30% following UAE.

For women with multiple fibroids who desire future pregnancy, outcomes are better after myomectomy than UAE. Compared to myomectomy, pregnancies after UAE have a higher incidence of preterm delivery and fetal malpresentation, and a higher trend for maternal postpartum hemorrhage and spontaneous abortion. These problems during pregnancy after UAE are not surprising, since embolization particles remain in the uterus and may affect normal uterine blood flow, and the fibroids remain in utero, albeit with a reduced volume. Nevertheless, subsequent pregnancy is not contraindicated for a woman who has undergone UAE for fibroids.

Cramping is expected in almost all women after embolization. Most require overnight hospitalization for pain control, and postprocedural pain lasts over 2 weeks in 5–10% patients. Approximately 33% of women experience fever, usually low grade. More severe "postembolization syndrome" may occur and is recognized by fever, leukocytosis, nausea, vomiting, malaise, anorexia, and abdominal pain. Approximately 15% of women require hospital readmission after UAE. More serious side effects include severe postembolization syndrome that requires hysterectomy. Hysterectomy might also be necessary for treatment failures. Since a histologic diagnosis is not obtained for UAE, there have been reports of delayed diagnosis of leiomyosarcoma. The embolization particles may occasionally enter the ovarian vasculature, and ovarian failure after UAE has been reported in 1–2% of women. Submucous myomas can dislodge and be expulsed vaginally in a sometimes painful process. A few deaths have been reported. Contraindications to UAE include pelvic infection or pelvic inflammatory disease, renal insufficiency, asymptomatic fibroids, or suspicion of cancer, and desire for future pregnancy is a relative contraindication.

Uterine vascular occlusion

Gynecologic surgeons have explored uterine vascular occlusion as an alternative to UAE. In most techniques, the uterine vessels are occluded at the time of laparoscopy and the fibroids are left to degenerate. While most of these techniques require laparoscopy and general anesthesia, and therefore are more invasive than UAE, the procedure provides an alternative approach to treating fibroids, with early reports describing outcomes similar to UAE. However, if a laparoscopic surgery is performed, it is reasonable to question the utility of choosing laparoscopic uterine vessel occlusion over the more established approach of laparoscopic myomectomy. More studies are needed before this approach is an accepted treatment for symptomatic uterine fibroids.

Myolysis

Myolysis was popularized as a laparoscopic treatment of uterine fibroids in the 1980s and 1990s, but has mostly been abandoned in favor of laparoscopic myomectomy. The technique was simple, and involved passing a monopolar or bipolar needle into the fibroid and then activating the current to destroy the tissue. This approach was successful in reducing fibroid size and improving symptoms, but multiple serosal punctures were required to treat each fibroid, adhesions often formed postoperatively, and although the fibroid became smaller it was not removed, as can be accomplished with laparoscopic myomectomy. Studies are needed to determine if an ultrasound-guided transvaginal myolysis needle can accomplish symptomatic relief in a less invasive approach than laparoscopy.

Magnetic resonance-guided focused ultrasound surgery

Magnetic resonance-guided focused ultrasound surgery (MRgFUS) was approved by the U.S. Food and Drug Administration for the treatment of symptomatic uterine fibroids in 2004, and more than 3,000 women worldwide had undergone this treatment for fibroids by 2007. MRgFUS utilizes MRI to provide a three-dimensional view of the uterus and fibroid, and allows for precise focusing of ultrasound energy to the fibroid, within a desired volume. MRI provides quantitative, real-time, thermal images of the treated area, and this ensures that the temperature generated is sufficient to cause heat ablation of the fibroid. MRgFUS has the great appeal that it is a nonsurgical approach, performed under sedation. Patient satisfaction is high, even though initial studies only showed approximately a 14% reduction in fibroid volume. The approach is expensive, requires approximately 3 hours of time dedicated in an MRI machine, and is too new to accumulate long-term follow-up data.

One possible limitation of this approach, compared to UAE, is that the energy is focused at the center of the fibroids, which is less well perfused and probably mitotically less active than the periphery, whereas UAE treats the vascular periphery of the fibroid. Few pregnancies have been reported after MRgFUS, but one study showed a live birth rate of only 40% of women who conceived after this treatment.

Until MRgFUS is more widely available and better long-term data are available, this approach should not be routinely recommended for women with symptomatic fibroids.

Hysterectomy

Hysterectomy is the only permanent treatment for symptomatic fibroids but should be reserved for the woman who has completed childbearing and is an appropriate surgical candidate. Hysterectomy may be most appealing to women who have suffered from symptomatic fibroids for many years, or who have attempted more conservative measures. Hysterectomy should not be considered for a woman who would consider having children in the future unless no other options are appropriate. Furthermore, hysterectomy should not be used in an asymptomatic woman with fibroids, regardless of the size of the uterus, unless cancer is suspected or visceral organs are compromised by ureteral obstruction due to fibroids.

The first recorded hysterectomy was performed in 120 AD by Soranus of Ephesus, and the first abdominal hysterectomy was described in 1843 by Heath in Manchester, United Kingdom. Approximately 600,000 hysterectomies are performed annually in the United States, and 200,000 of those are for fibroids, the leading indication for hysterectomy.

Hysterectomy can be performed as an open procedure (abdominal hysterectomy), vaginal hysterectomy, laparoscopic-assisted vaginal hysterectomy, or total laparoscopic hysterectomy. If the cervix is preserved, the procedure is considered "supracervical," and removal of the cervix and uterus is a "total" hysterectomy. As fibroids may recur in the cervix after a subtotal hysterectomy, a total hysterectomy is most commonly performed. The type of surgery should be chosen based on the characteristics of the fibroids, the presence of other abnormalities such as pelvic adhesions or ovarian cysts, and the technical skills of the surgeon. Safety and outcome are the primary factors in choosing the approach. When these are equal, the procedure that provides the fastest return to full recovery should be used. Usually, recovery is shortest with uncomplicated vaginal hysterectomy, and then laparoscopic hysterectomy, followed by laparoscopic-assisted vaginal hysterectomy, and abdominal hysterectomy.

The size of the uterus and location of the fibroids can pose a special problem during hysterectomy. Regardless of the technique chosen, selective myomectomy can help improve exposure and simplify the surgical approach. Additionally, during vaginal hysterectomy, the uterus can be wedged or divided after the uterine vasculature has been occluded and cut. Advances in instrumentation, especially the use of vessel-sealing clamps and special devices for morcellation, have increased the use of laparoscopic hysterectomy for fibroids.

Adenomyosis

Adenomyosis is a condition in which endometrial glands are present in the myometrium. The etiology of adenomyosis is unclear, but since it often occurs in women who have been pregnant or have undergone uterine instrumentation, most cases probably arise when the endometrium is dislodged into the myometrium. Typical symptoms of adenomyosis include progressive menorrhagia, dysmenorrhea, and, in some cases, menometrorrhagia. Adenomyosis may coincide with endometriosis, and some women experience dyspareunia, infertility, or chronic pelvic pain. As with uterine fibroids, the peak incidence of adenomyosis is found in women between the ages of 35 and 50. Both conditions improve after menopause. The adenomyosis tissue is hormonally responsive, and can proliferate, mature, and bleed in response to ovarian hormones, concurrent with the changes in the endometrium. Adenomyosis can be focal or diffuse, and is sometimes difficult to distinguish from fibroids by ultrasound (see Figure 7.1 above). MRI may help to establish the diagnosis, but should only be ordered if identification of adenomyosis would alter patient care (Figure 7.8).

Medical management

Adenomyosis is hormonally sensitive and in most cases responds well to hormone therapy. If pain is not controlled with nonsteroidal anti-inflammatory drugs (NSAIDs), hormonal contraception can reduce bleeding and pain in

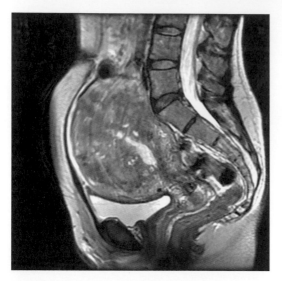

Figure 7.8 Magnetic resonance imaging showing adenomyosis.

most women, but hormone use preclude pregnancy during treatment. In many women, NSAIDs such as ibuprofen 400–800 mg or naproxen 275–550 mg provide satisfactory relief of dysmenorrhea and may reduce menstrual bleeding.

If the patient is not interested in conceiving, treatment options include continuous or cyclic oral contraceptives, the contraceptive patch, and the contraceptive ring. If pain is not relieved with hormonal contraception, continuous high-dose progestin therapy can be effective, such as medroxyprogesterone acetate 30 mg daily, norethindrone 5 mg daily initially and increased by 2.5 mg until menses stops, or megestrol acetate 40 mg daily. If progestin therapy resolves symptoms and is tolerated well, the patient can change to depot medroxyprogesterone acetate 150 mg administered intramuscularly every 3 months.

Alternately, the levonorgestrel progestin IUD (Mirena) has been shown to reduce menorrhagia and dysmenorrhea. This approach provides several advantages over other hormonal therapy, primarily because of its simplicity after placement. Its low systemic absorption of hormones leads to fewer side effects than with other types of hormonal contraception. Once placed, the IUD is effective for 5 years.

Unfortunately, just as the uterine endometrium resumes normal function after discontinuation of hormonal contraception, adenomyosis and associated symptoms recur quickly. Surgical options are limited by the diffuse nature of the condition, and hysterectomy is the only permanent cure. As with fibroids, the type of surgery should be determined by safety first, and if more than one procedure is equally safe, the procedure that allows the fastest full recovery is most appropriate. Other interventional approaches are less successful for adenomyosis, including UAE and conservative resection of the adenomyosis. Treatment failure rate is higher after UAE for adenomyosis than for fibroids, although some find this option attractive as a "last chance" approach before hysterectomy. With the exception of a focal adenomyoma, conservative resection of adenomyosis is difficult. The diffuse nature of adenomyosis obscures the margin between myometrium and adenomyosis, and once an incision has been made the remaining tissue is fragile and the incision can be difficult or impossible to close properly. As a result, surgical resection of diffuse adenomyosis should be avoided, if possible.

Conclusions

Accurate diagnosis allows the most appropriate option to be offered. The selected treatment should provide the greatest relief of symptoms with the least risk. When surgery is indicated, the practitioner should choose the safest procedure. If more than one option provides comparable safety, the procedure with the fastest recovery should be used.

Selected bibliography

Antibiotic prophylaxis for gynecologic procedures. ACOG Practice Bulletin No. 104. American College of Obstetricians and Gynecologists. Obstet Gynecol 2009;113:1180–9.

Bosteels J, Weyers S, Puttemans P et al. The effectiveness of hysteroscopy in improving pregnancy rates in subfertile women without other gynaecological symptoms: a systematic review. Hum Reprod Update 2010;16:1–11.

Broder MS, Goodwin S, Chen G et al. Comparison of long-term outcomes of myomectomy and uterine artery embolization. Obstet Gynecol 2002;100:864–8.

Ferrazzi E, Zupi E, Leone FP et al. How often are endometrial polyps malignant in asymptomatic postmenopausal women? A multicenter study. Am J Obstet Gynecol 2009;200:235. e1–6.

Goldberg, J, Pereira L, Berghella V et al. Pregnancy outcomes after treatment for fibromyomata: uterine artery embolization versus laparoscopic myomectomy. Am J Obstet Gynecol 2004;191:18–21.

Hodge JC, Morton CC. Genetic heterogeneity among uterine leiomyomata: insights into malignant progression. Hum Mol Genet 2007;16(Spec. No. 1):R7–13.

Hurst BS, Matthews ML, Marshburn PB. Laparoscopic myomectomy for symptomatic uterine myomas. Fertil Steril 2005;83:1–23.

Hurst BS, Stackhouse DJ, Matthews ML, Marshburn PB. Uterine artery embolization for symptomatic uterine myomas. Fertil Steril 2000;74:855–69.

Lasmar RB, Dias R, Barrozo PR, Oliveira MA, Coutinho Eda S, da Rosa DB. Prevalence of hysteroscopic findings and histologic diagnoses in patients with abnormal uterine bleeding. Fertil Steril 2008;89:1803–7.

Practice Committee of American Society for Reproductive Medicine. Indications and options for endometrial ablation. Fertil Steril 2008;90:S236–40.

Rabinovici J, David M, Fukunishi H, Morita Y, Gostout BS, Stewart EA, MRgFUS Study Group. Pregnancy outcome after magnetic resonance-guided focused ultrasound surgery (MRgFUS) for conservative treatment of uterine fibroids. Fertil Steril 2010;93:199–209.

Sheiner E, Bashiri A, Levy A, Hershkovitz R, Katz M, Mazor M. Obstetric characteristics and perinatal outcome of pregnancies with uterine leiomyomas. J Reprod Med 2004;49:182–6.

Shozu M, Murakami K, Inoue M. Aromatase and leiomyoma of the uterus. Sem Reprod Med 2004;22:51–60.

Sunkara SK, Khairy M, El-Toukhy T, Khalaf Y, Coomarasamy A. The effect of intramural fibroids without uterine cavity involvement on the outcome of IVF treatment: a systematic review and meta-analysis. Hum Reprod 2010;25:418–29.

Waddell G, Desindes S, Takser L, Beauchemin MC, Bessette P. Cervical ripening using vaginal misoprostol before hysteroscopy: a double-blind randomized trial. J Minim Invas Gynecol 2008;15:739–44.

Walocha JA, Litwin JA, Miodonski AJ. Vascular system of intramural leiomyomata revealed by corrosion casting and scanning electron microscopy. Hum Reprod 2003;18:1088–93.

8

Infrequent Menstrual Bleeding and Amenorrhea During the Reproductive Years

Paul B. Miller

Greenville Hospital System, Greenville, South Carolina, USA

Introduction

The approach to patients who present with menstrual disorders during the reproductive years (i.e., from menarche at age 13 to menopause at age 51) starts with a consideration of two physiologic compartments: the endocrine system and the urogenital tract.

> **⚛ SCIENCE REVISITED**
>
> Within the endocrine system, the interplay between the hypothalamus, pituitary, and ovaries depends upon a delicate balance of events, each sequentially feeding back to the central nervous system as the control center of reproductive function. The proper balance and sequential production of the sex steroid hormones estrogen and progesterone is required for adequate endometrial proliferation, secretory transformation, and later shedding at the time of menses. The development and shedding of the endometrium is in turn dependent on not just the hormonal signals from the ovaries, but also the presence of a functionally responsive uterine cavity with a normal outflow tract. Any irregularities in these areas can lead to the absence of menses (amenorrhea) or prolonged intervals between menses (oligomenorrhea).

Amenorrhea is typically designated as primary or secondary. Women with primary amenorrhea have never undergone menarche and may or may not have any development of secondary sexual characteristics. In the absence of secondary sexual characteristics, formal evaluation of primary amenorrhea should begin by age 14; otherwise, initiation of testing should begin by age 16 if the patient does have normal pubertal progression. Since a complete discussion of primary amenorrhea entails a review of the various causes of pubertal delay, the reader is referred to Chapter 3 for more information. A widely used working definition of secondary amenorrhea is the absence of menses for 6 months or the equivalent duration of three menstrual cycles. Of course, from a practical standpoint, one need not wait for either of these conditions to occur depending on the clinical circumstances. A prime example is implementation of a urine pregnancy test for a woman who is even a few days delayed for menses if she usually has regular cycles. Oligomenorrhea may be regular or irregular, but is most often associated with an intermenstrual interval of greater than 35 days. Using these definitions clinically will help practitioners avoid hasty evaluations and aid in educating and counseling patients.

In an otherwise healthy reproductive-aged population, the expected incidence of secondary amenorrhea is 3–4%, although the number of affected women with disorders such as polycystic

Disorders of Menstruation, 1st edition. Edited by Paul B. Marshburn and Bradley S. Hurst.
© 2011 Blackwell Publishing Ltd.

Table 8.1 Common causes of secondary amenorrhea

Category	Frequency (%)
Low or normal FSH	66
• Weight loss/anorexia • Hypothalamic dysfunction • Chronic anovulation/PCOS • Hypothyroidism • Cushing syndrome • Pituitary tumor, empty sella • Sheehan syndrome	
Gonadal failure—high FSH	12
• 46,XX • Abnormal karyotype	
Hyperprolactinemia	13
Anatomic	7
• Asherman syndrome	
Hyperandrogenism	2
• Ovarian tumor • Congenital adrenal hyperplasia • Idiopathic	

FSH, follicle-stimulating hormone; PCOS, polycystic ovarian syndrome.
Reproduced from Reindollar et al, 1986, with permission.

ovary syndrome (PCOS) appears to be increasing. The corresponding rate for oligomenorrhea is difficult to estimate since women will quite often have transient periods of oligomenorrhea before becoming frankly amenorrheic or eumenorrheic. For this reason, it is best to consider the progression of eumenorrhea to amenorrhea as a continuum, with oligomenorrhea somewhere between the extremes. Likewise, during the discussion of the etiology, evaluation, and treatment of amenorrhea that follows, one can often infer that oligomenorrheic women suffer from similar causes of their disorder, albeit to a lesser extent. A review of 262 women who presented to a tertiary care center with a chief complaint of secondary amenorrhea reported frequencies of diagnoses seen in Table 8.1.

History and physical examination

A detailed history and physical examination are essential to directing further investigation of a woman presenting with amenorrhea (Figure 8.1). Documentation of age at menarche, periodicity of menses, intermenstrual interval, and date of the last menstrual period are requisite starting points. Likewise, enquiring about recent medical problems, procedures, and medications will often reveal proximate causes for menstrual disturbances. A menstrual calendar and documentation of any changes in weight are also helpful in the evaluation of these patients.

Documentation of skin changes including hirsutism or acne can provide evidence for PCOS. Fatigue, hot or cold intolerance, or a history of breast discharge should be documented, raising suspicions about hyperprolactinemia or thyroid disease. The presence of vasomotor symptoms may be the only noticeable change other than irregular menses for women entering the menopausal transition period. Patients should always be queried regarding exercise and dietary habits, as obsessive behavior in either area may be a sign

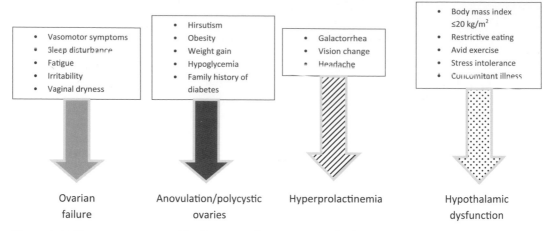

Figure 8.1 Diagnoses suggested by history and examination findings.

of an eating disorder and subsequent hypothalamic dysfunction. Moreover, any recent stressful events noted in the social history should provoke a higher suspicion of a hypothalamic disorder. Eliciting a thorough family history may reveal pervasive problems with obesity, metabolic syndrome, or diabetes, all of which may be associated with ovulatory dysfunction and menstrual irregularity. One may also discover a familial pattern of premature menopause that inherently increases the patient's own risk for gonadal failure.

On physical examination, signs of change in hormonally sensitive areas outside the genital tract (e.g., facial hair, baldness, breast development) are important to document, along with body mass index (weight in kilograms divided by height in meters squared). Women at either extreme of body mass index (i.e., very thin or obese) increase their risk of ovulatory dysfunction. Changes in hair or skin (e.g., brittle hair, thick and dry skin, hand and face edema) may be signs of hypothyroidism. Galactorrhea, or milky breast discharge, may be a manifestation of hyperprolactinemia, from either a functional adenoma or other pituitary tumor. Anyone suspected of hyperprolactinemia also deserves a fundoscopic examination to assess for papilledema that can occur with vascular compression from a large pituitary tumor. Obese women may have evidence of acanthosis nigricans along skin creases at the base of the neck and in the axilla (Figure 8.2), indicative of insulin resistance and possible diabetes.

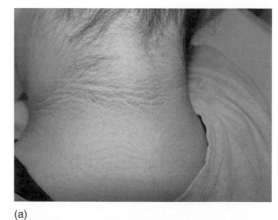
(a)

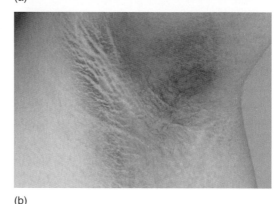
(b)

Figure 8.2 Acanthosis nigricans of (a) the neck and (b) the axilla. Reproduced from (a) www.fromyourdoctor.com and (b) webmd.com (see Plate 8.2).

Regarding the genital tract, examination of the external genitalia should include assessment of hair patterns and any evidence of virilization (e.g., clitoromegaly, deepening of the voice, temporal balding, increased muscle mass). Patency of the vagina should be noted, along with the presence of a normal cervix and cervical os. Normal vaginal rugation and moisture are important signs of adequate estrogenization of genital tissues and may help to eliminate cases of gonadal failure. Establishing the presence of a normal, patent external cervical os lessens the potential for outflow obstruction due to stenosis or congenital anomaly. The presence of a mass on pelvic examination can also direct the evaluation of the amenorrheic women, as ovarian neoplasia (e.g., granulosa cell tumors) can occasionally create a hormonal milieu associated with absent or infrequent menses.

Further patient evaluation

After first testing for pregnancy with a urine or serum human chorionic gonadotropin (hCG) assay, initial laboratory investigation should include measurement of serum thyrotropin (TSH) and prolactin levels (Figure 8.3). Although they are not the most common causes of amenorrhea, both hypothyroidism and hyperprolactinemia are easily treated, with a near-immediate response to adequate therapy.

✷ TIPS & TRICKS

Hyperprolactinemia can be associated with hypothyroidism. Stimulation of prolactin-secreting pituitary cells can be caused by thyrotropin-releasing hormone (which drives thyroid-stimulating hormone [TSH] elevation), which will be increased in most cases of hypothyroidism. For that reason, TSH levels should be determined along with prolactin levels if galactorrhea or hyperprolactinemia is discovered. If TSH *is* elevated, correction of hypothyroidism with levothyroxine treatment should be instituted first. If correction of hypothyroidism does not normalize elevated prolactin levels, further evaluation is warranted.

Women with either hypo- or hyperthyroidism may exhibit ovulatory dysfunction ranging from amenorrhea to menorrhagia. Patients with hyperprolactinemia, depending on the level of aberrant prolactin secretion, may have subtle menstrual changes such as late luteal spotting, all the way to frank amenorrhea and hypoestrogenism. Other laboratory tests that are worthwhile include estradiol, follicle-stimulating hormone (FSH), and in some cases luteinizing hormone (LH). The latter may be particularly helpful in amenorrhea secondary to hypothalamic dysfunction where FSH and estradiol levels are often within normal limits. Physical examination evidence of hyperandrogenism requires screening for hyperandrogenemia with serum testosterone and dehydroepiandrosterone sulfate levels.

✋ CAUTION!

A word of caution is in order when interpreting the results of the initial laboratory investigation. The practitioner needs to understand that a single serum sample represents a snapshot in time of what is a dynamic ebb and flow of circulating hormones. Some hormones, including cortisol and prolactin, exhibit diurnal rhythms as well, while others, including progesterone, estrogen, and the gonadotropins, change radically during a normal menstrual cycle. For example, fluctuations in estradiol levels for perimenopausal women may lead to the false conclusion that their vasomotor symptoms are not related to estrogen withdrawal, when in fact they may have a tremendous variation in serum levels throughout the day. Stated differently, a test result that lies within the established normal range for a particular assay does not eliminate the possibility that the overall hormonal milieu is off balance. Repeated or further testing is required in such cases to minimize the risk of either over- or undertreating the patient.

After establishing by either blood or urine testing for the beta subunit of hCG that the patient is not pregnant, an assessment of a woman's estrogen status is warranted. Traditionally, a progestin (e.g., medroxyprogesterone acetate 10 mg orally)

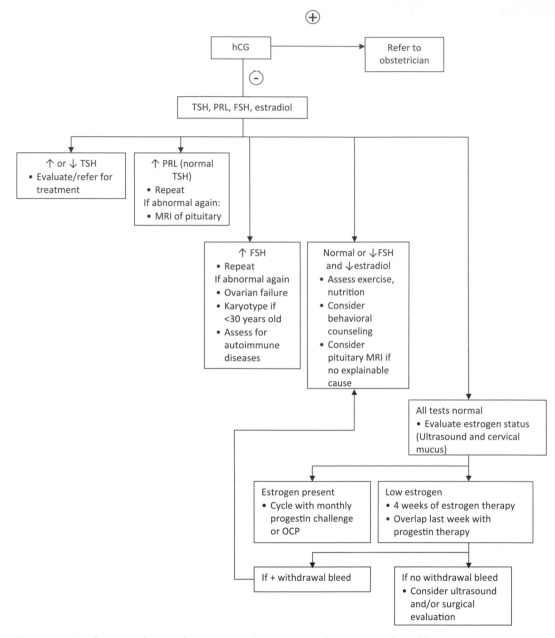

Figure 8.3 Evaluation of secondary amenorrhea. PRL, prolactin. For other abbreviations, see text.

or progesterone (e.g., 200 mg orally or vaginally for 10 days, or a single dose of 150 mg of progesterone in oil intramuscularly) has been administered to determine whether a woman has adequate estrogen to stimulate endometrial growth that will shed and bleed after withdrawal of the progestin. Withdrawal bleeding in response to exogenous progestin, however, was

found in 50% of women with hypergonadotropic hypogonadism (high FSH, low estradiol). Furthermore, some women with hyperandrogenism, chronic anovulation, and estrogen present (PCOS) may fail to have a withdrawal bleed secondary to an antiproliferative effect of androgens on the endometrium. Poor oral absorption of progestin medication could also be a reason for the absence of withdrawal bleeding after medication discontinuation.

For these reasons, practitioners are encouraged to use other clinical measures to determine whether a woman has an adequate level of estrogenization, such as the presence of thin, watery, clear, and profuse cervical mucus (Figure 8.4) and the presence of an endometrial thickness greater than 6 mm on ultrasound exam. In this manner, a woman may be saved the time, expense, and possible side effects of oral, vaginal, or intramuscular progestin administration. Correction of thyroid and prolactin abnormalities should be

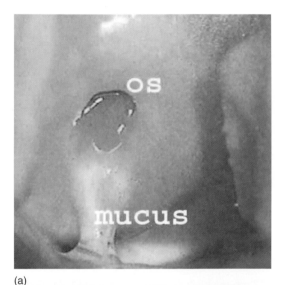

(a)

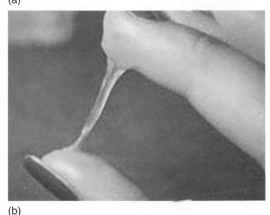

(b)

Figure 8.4 Estrogenized cervical mucus. Reproduced from (a) http://infertilitybooks.com and (b) http://commons.wikimedia.org (see Plate 8.4).

primarily identified and managed as discussed later in the chapter.

If a patient is deemed to have inadequate estrogen present (i.e., hypoestrogenism), attention should then focus on central defects in the pituitary and hypothalamus (hypogonadotropic hypogonadism) or to intrinsic ovarian failure (hypergonadotropic hypogonadism). The key to understanding which of these etiologies is at play is FSH: in cases of the former, FSH is usually in the low normal range or diminished; in cases of the latter, FSH is markedly elevated in the menopausal range, typically 40 IU/L or more.

In some cases of hypothalamic dysfunction or the menopausal transition, circulating estradiol levels fluctuate dramatically, making a single assay result of little predictive value. However, in more profound cases of hypothalamic dysfunction and after the menopausal transition, estradiol levels are typically low (≤30 pg/mL) and incapable of stimulating adequate endometrial proliferation. The exception is the obese patient who may be menopausal but maintains higher levels of estrogen from aromatase-mediated conversion of circulating androgens to estrogen in adipose cells. In cases of functional hypothalamic amenorrhea, FSH may be within normal limits; however, simultaneously measured LH levels are usually low, reflecting its shorter half-life (20 minutes) compared to FSH (4 hours). In rare circumstances, FSH and LH may both be within the normal range but lack sufficient bioactivity even though they are immunoreactive and show up in the laboratory assay. In contrast, in patients with gonadal failure, the feedback loop between hypothalamus, pituitary, and ovaries is disrupted, leading to loss of estrogen negative feedback on the brain and a subsequent elevation in both pituitary FSH and LH secretion.

When gonadotropin and estradiol levels are within normal limits (i.e., eugonadotropic amenorrhea), suspicion rises for failure of end-organ response and outflow obstruction. Transvaginal ultrasound of the uterus will most often give the best determination of the presence or absence of functional endometrium. The appearance of an endometrial thickness of 6 mm or greater (especially if a trilaminar appearance is present; see Chapter 6) suggests functional endometrium, while a thin 2 mm endometrial stripe with an echogenic appearance is often associated with endometrial scarring or atrophy.

A trial of exogenous estrogen and progestin may be warranted as the next step if the ultrasound determination is equivocal. Most regimens used for this purpose include estrogen alone for 3 weeks (e.g., oral conjugated equine estrogens 1.25 mg or estradiol 2 mg daily, transdermal estradiol patch 0.1 mg twice weekly) followed by a fourth week of estrogen accompanied by a daily dose of progestin (e.g., oral medroxyprogesterone acetate 10 mg or micronized progesterone 200 mg) or a single intramuscular injection of progesterone in oil 150–200 mg. These doses should adequately stimulate endometrial proliferation and secretory transformation followed by menstrual shedding as estrogen and progesterone levels fall. Absence of bleeding after such a 1-month regimen implies that there is a lack of functional endometrium, or that the cervix, vagina, or endometrial cavity is obstructed.

In cases of primary amenorrhea, congenital anomalies such as an imperforate hymen, transverse vaginal septum, and vaginal and cervical agenesis are part of the differential diagnosis at this point. Typically, these conditions would exhibit signs and symptoms of cryptomenorrhea (hidden menses) with cyclic lower abdominal pain (see Chapter 3). These diagnoses would not, however, apply to anyone presenting with secondary amenorrhea.

For those women who have had normal menses in the past, the prospect of scarring and the formation of intrauterine synechiae (Asherman syndrome) is also a possible diagnosis. The typical history of a woman with this condition includes vigorous curettage of an infected uterus such as one sees with second-trimester abortions with retained placental fragments following delivery. Cervical stenosis is rare in the absence of some sort of trauma, such as a loop electrosurgical excision procedure (LEEP) or cryotherapy for dysplasia. Vaginal stricture to the point of closure may occur with trauma of one sort or another but is virtually unheard of in the absence of hypoestrogenism.

If hypogonadotropic hypogonadism is confirmed, imaging of the hypothalamic/pituitary region is the last step to exclude any potentially treatable abnormality. In most centers, the greatest sensitivity is achieved with a focused magnetic resonance imaging (MRI) scan with a specific request for close assessment of the pituitary area. Ordering a simple head radiograph called a coned-down view of the sella turcica does not offer the interpreting radiologist enough information to focus in on potential diagnoses.

☆ TIPS & TRICKS

Mention of the patient's clinical condition and the presence or absence of hyperprolactinemia increase the pretest probability of finding a significant lesion to explain the abnormality. Occasionally, lesions outside the sella turcica can cause compression of the pituitary stalk leading to hyperprolactinemia or pituitary dysfunction. Such tumors are important to document as they can sometimes be malignant and threaten the patient's health.

Hypothalamic and pituitary causes of amenorrhea

Adequate pulsatile release of gonadotropin-releasing hormone (GnRH) from the hypothalamus into the portal circulation relies upon multiple inputs from other areas of the brain. Endogenous opioids, neurotransmitters, peptides, and steroids all feed back on centers controlling GnRH secretion, making a precise diagnosis of altered pulsatility an exercise in endocrine and paracrine theory.

There is no practical means for measuring GnRH pulses in a clinical setting. What one does see is a hormonal milieu similar to that of young, prepubertal girls prior to complete maturation of their hypothalamic–pituitary–ovarian axes: notably, FSH is low or more often low-normal with an FSH:LH ratio of two or more. Estradiol, prolactin, and TSH are usually within normal limits, but at the lower end of the normal range. Often women will experience surges in LH activity that in turn lead to increased thecal androgen secretion and overt manifestations of androgen excess such as acne. Some authors have likened it to a "second puberty" since women with hypothalamic dysfunction have the same hormonal fluctuations and oligo-/anovulation that are typically seen in normal young teens.

All women with the clinical diagnosis of functional hypothalamic amenorrhea require further questioning regarding their levels of stress, exercise, and nutrition since obsessive behaviors in any of these areas may be the root of their menstrual problem. Difficulty arises, however, in judging how much is too much in each of these areas. In general, patients who report stress-related sleep disorders on a regular basis, strained relationships at work or at home due to stress, or neglect of personal health or fitness due to overwork may benefit from stress counseling. To this end, remarkable strides have been made with mind–body techniques that allow patients to elicit an equally potent relaxation response to combat innate stress responses throughout the day. Techniques such as cognitive behavioral therapy, meditation, and mindfulness lower heart rate and blood pressure, improve sleep, and aid in prevention of immune dysfunction and cardiovascular disease.

Assessment of exercise habits becomes tricky given the many salutary effects of physical fitness balanced against chronic states of negative energy balance and altered levels of neurotransmitters. During exercise, levels of endogenous opioids increase dramatically, along with levels of stress hormones such as cortisol and norepinephrine (noradrenaline), leading to suppression of the GnRH pulse generator in the hypothalamus.

⬡ SCIENCE REVISITED

Leptin is a protein produced in adipocytes that is involved in the regulation of satiety and hunger at the level of the hypothalamus. In normal circumstances, leptin plays a permissive role in reproduction by signaling the central nervous system that enough stored energy exists in the periphery to sustain the metabolic demands of a pregnancy. As the percentage of body fat decreases, so does leptin expression. If leptin levels decrease, pulsatile gonadotropin releasing hormone secretion will be dampened, leading to poor hypothalamic signaling to the pituitary and subsequent hypogonadism.

Women with eating disorders are often secretive and may present with menstrual dysfunction as one of the earliest manifestations of disease. A thorough understanding of the *Diagnostic and Statistical Manual of Mental Disorders* IV (DSM-IV) criteria for eating disorders aids in the expeditious diagnosis and treatment of women prior to any serious metabolic derangements that could affect other organ systems. The DSM-IV criteria for diagnosing anorexia nervosa are:

- refusal to maintain weight within a normal range for height and age (more than 15% below ideal body weight);
- fear of weight gain;
- severe body image disturbance in which body image is the predominant measure of self-worth; with denial of the seriousness of the illness;
- in postmenarchal females, absence of the menstrual cycle or amenorrhea (for longer than three cycles).

The DSM-IV criteria for bulimia nervosa are:

- episodes of binge eating with a sense of loss of control;
- binge-eating being followed by compensatory behavior of the purging type (self-induced vomiting, laxative abuse, diuretic abuse) or nonpurging type (excessive exercise, fasting, or strict diets);
- binges and the resulting compensatory behavior must occur a minimum of two times per week for 3 months;
- dissatisfaction with body shape and weight.

Other causes of secondary hypothalamic amenorrhea are much less common and are generally more readily apparent after eliciting a proper history and following a stepwise diagnostic algorithm. Infectious causes such as tuberculosis and syphilis are detectable with skin testing and serology, and are rare in Western societies. Encephalitis, meningitis, and sarcoidosis have all been associated with hypothalamic dysfunction. Likewise, women with chronic diseases (e.g., renal failure, diabetes, malignancy) often present with amenorrhea due to the body's ability to shut down nonessential functions such as reproduction in order to allow more energy for fighting the more life-threatening problem. Central nervous system neoplasms (craniopharyngioma, germinoma, hamartoma, Langerhans cell histiocytosis, teratoma, endodermal sinus tumor, metastatic carcinoma; Figure 8.5) may directly affect hypothalamic/pituitary signaling by disrupting neural pathways, or may alter portal circulation, thereby preventing the stimulation of pituitary cells by their respective releasing factors. In cases of the latter, prolactin is elevated due to its chronic inhibition by dopamine secreted from the hypothalamus. Often these conditions are accompanied by significant constitutional signs and symptoms such as severe headache or cranial nerve abnormalities.

Hyperprolactinemia

Pituitary adenomas, with the exception of prolactin-secreting adenomas, are relatively uncommon causes of secondary amenorrhea. As many as one third of women with no identifiable cause of secondary amenorrhea will have hyperprolactinemia. Importantly, serum prolactin must be measured in more than one sample several days apart due to a large number of physiologic conditions that can cause transient elevation (Table 8.2), thus leading to misdiagnosis. Simultaneous measurement of TSH is also required because patients with primary hypothyroidism and elevated TSH also have elevations in thyroid-releasing hormone from the hypothalamus. The latter is a potent stimulator of prolactin secretion that need not be measured as long as a reliable TSH assay is available. Likewise, numerous medications can stimulate prolactin release and should be excluded as potential confounding sources (Table 8.3).

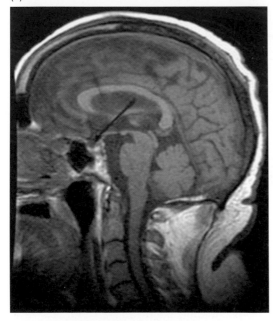

(a)

(b)

Figure 8.5 Magnetic resonance imaging scan of (a) a prolactin-secreting adenoma and (b) empty sella syndrome. Reproduced from (a) http://kibbeyctprocedures.blogspot.com and (b) http://www.radgray.com.

Table 8.2 Physiologic causes of hyperprolactinemia

Nipple stimulation
Stress
Intercourse
Sleep
Exercise
Seizures
Hypothyroidism
Hepatic failure
Renal failure
Lung and renal carcinoma
Ovarian teratoma
Uterine fibroids

Table 8.3 Medications that may cause hyperprolactinemia

Antipsychotics (neuroleptics)
• Phenothiazines
• Thioxanthenes
• Butyrophenones
• Atypical antipsychotics
Antidepressants
• Tricyclic and tetracyclic antidepressants
• Monoamine oxidase inhibitors
• Selective serotonin reuptake inhibitors
• Other
Opiates and cocaine
Antihypertensive medications
• Verapamil
• Methyldopa
• Reserpine
Gastrointestinal medications
• Metoclopramide
• Domperidone
• Histamine-2 receptor blockers
Protease inhibitors
Estrogens

A contentious issue arises when a patient who is dependent on a prolactin seretagog to maintain health and wellbeing also wishes to conceive but has oligo/amenorrhea. In such cases, alternative medical regimens should be discussed with the patient and her prescribing physician before starting her on prolactin-lowering medications. In some circumstances, simply lowering the dose of medication may be enough to improve menstrual and ovulatory function. It should be understood that prolactin has a suppressive effect on hypothalamic signaling to the pituitary that follows a continuum as levels rise. Therefore, with mild hyperprolactinemia, patients may simply experience luteal phase deficiency characterized by late luteal spotting or short luteal phase length. As levels rise, dysfunction progresses to oligomenorrhea with diminished integrated serum estrogen production throughout the cycle, followed by amenorrhea and eventual hypoestrogenism.

Pituitary imaging is warranted in any case of persistent hyperprolactinemia that does not correct after eliminating all potential causes. Imaging recommendations based on threshold levels of prolactin (e.g., ≥50 ng/mL) fail to account for nonadenomatous lesions that may compress the pituitary stalk and adenomatous lesions that co-secrete prolactin, such as growth hormone-secreting tumors. The latter are often associated with only modest elevations in prolactin that may not meet threshold criteria, potentially delaying diagnosis if overlooked.

MRI is the modality of choice for evaluation of the hypothalamus and pituitary. Once detected, adenomas are classified based on their size, with lesions less than 10 mm being designated microadenomas and those 10 mm or more being designated macroadenomas.

> **☞ CAUTION!**
>
> Patients with prolactin-secreting macroadenomas may need to be referred for a formal visual field evaluation. Extension of a pituitary adenoma above the sella turcica may cause compression of the optic chiasm resulting in "tunnel vision" (bitemporal hemianopsia). Prior to treatment of prolactin-secreting macroadenomas, it may also be appropriate to proceed with a neurosurgery consultation. Rarely will treatment of a prolactin-secreting macroadenoma with a dopamine agonist (bromocriptine, cabergoline) cause rapid tumor regression and bleeding into the tumor. If this happens (pituitary apoplexy), emergency neurosurgical assistance may be needed.

Fewer than 5% of microadenomas will grow to become macroadenomas, with as many as one third spontaneously regressing without treatment. Prolactin-secreting adenomas account for the vast majority of adenomas and are considered benign lesions, as histologic examination reveals normal hormone-producing cells without evidence of atypia or malignancy.

Both micro- and macroadenomas generally respond to treatment with dopamine agonists such as bromocriptine and cabergoline.

> ## ✋ CAUTION!
>
> Bromocriptine has been used for many years as a first-line therapy for management of prolactin-secreting adenomas. The medication must be started with low doses initially and should be taken once or twice daily. Bromocriptine administration may be associated with undesirable side effects (e.g., nausea, hypotension, dizziness, headache). Cabergoline is a long-acting dopamine agonist that may be administered one or two times weekly with excellent suppression of prolactin secretion and fewer side effects. Recent evidence suggests that the high doses of this medication used for Parkinson disease patients may cause valvular heart disease. Low doses (0.25–0.5 mg once or twice weekly), however, such as those used to treat hyperprolactinemia, have not been similarly implicated.

Transsphenoidal surgery is reserved for recalcitrant cases only since the long-term cure rate is only approximately 50% depending on the size of the tumor, and the risk for panhypopituitarism is substantial (10–30%).

Several special cases of hyperprolactinemia deserve inclusion in the differential diagnosis of secondary amenorrhea. The first is a condition known as empty sella syndrome, in which a defect in the sellar diaphragm allows extension of the subarachnoid space into the pituitary fossa. The compressed pituitary oversecretes prolactin, leading to oligo/amenorrhea. Other adenomatous growths may be present in empty sella syndrome, necessitating the need for annual surveillance for this benign condition. The second special case of hyperprolactinemia is the idiopathic variety in which pituitary imaging fails to detect any abnormalities. Up to one third of these patients will resolve spontaneously, with only 10% progressing to have microadenomas. Idiopathic cases are best treated as microadenomas when the size is below the threshold of detection by conventional means.

Ovulatory dysfunction and polycystic ovaries

Although a complete review of ovulatory dysfunction and polycystic ovaries is found in Chapter 5, it bears mentioning that the most common cause of oligo/amenorrhea for non-pregnant women in the reproductive years is failed ovulation. The classic example of an anovulatory woman (obese, hirsute, amenorrheic) is one end of a spectrum of disease that involves multiple organ systems. It is important for caregivers to realize that 20% of women with polycystic ovaries based on standardized criteria are nonobese and that they quite often do ovulate, albeit at irregular intervals. Any patient with irregular menses and hirsutism should be suspected of having polycystic ovaries regardless of laboratory testing.

In fact, serum hormone levels can be misleading since gonadotropins may fluctuate and estrogen levels are typically normal. Androgen levels may also be normal, although free androgen levels are frequently elevated due to high levels of LH-stimulated androgen production in the face of diminished production of sex hormone-binding globulin (SHBG). The latter is a regulatory protein that along with albumin binds 98–99% of circulating testosterone in women. Insulin resistance and subsequent hyperinsulinemia, hallmarks of PCOS, lead to decreased hepatic production of SHBG.

Treatment for chronic anovulation involves the use of cyclic progestin therapy to induce withdrawal menses (e.g., medroxyprogesterone acetate 10 mg orally for 7–10 days every month) or suppressive therapy with oral contraceptive pills (OCPs) in a traditional cyclic or continuous active pattern (active pills only for 9–12 weeks). Hormonal therapies such as these prevent the development of endometrial hyperplasia and lower the risk for endometrial cancer. OCPs have a distinct advantage for PCOS patients with hirsutism in that they suppress ovarian steroidogenesis, thus decreasing estrogen and testosterone production. They also increase the hepatic production of SHBG, thereby decreasing the percentage of free testosterone in the circulation. Continuous active OCPs provide even tighter control of ovarian hormone production since they prevent a potential escape phenomenon for the ovaries during the 7 days of placebos in most pill packs. Further treatment of hyperandrogenism is addressed elsewhere in this text.

Hypergonadotropic hypogonadism

Women are born with a finite number of oocytes that undergo continuous waves of growth and atresia. As oocyte numbers decline over time, ovarian production of inhibins A and B from granulosa cells decreases, releasing FSH from tonic suppression. As a result, one sees a gradual increase in FSH levels in the early follicular phase (cycle day 3) for women in their late 30s, with an accelerated rise after 40 until menopause. At menopause, FSH levels exceed 40 mIU/mL and remain elevated on several occasions months apart.

Women who experience menopause prior to age 40 are said to have premature ovarian failure or primary ovarian insufficiency. For most women, age at menopause is genetically determined, so a thorough family history is in order for anyone presenting with the onset of amenorrhea prior to age 40. The vast majority of patients will present with hypoestrogenic symptoms such as hot flashes, mood swings, and vaginal dryness, which should immediately raise the suspicion of the menopausal transition or the menopausal state. A list of potential etiologies is found in Table 8.4. Taken as a whole, any condition that effects gonadal development in utero (e.g., gonadal dysgenesis) or accelerates loss of ovarian follicles, whether due to toxicity (e.g., chemotherapy) or surgery (e.g., oophorectomy in a child), may lead to early gonadal failure.

Special cases worth noting are gonadal dysgenesis and fragile X syndrome. Patients with a 45,X karyotype usually present in childhood with the typical phenotypic features of Turner syndrome (short stature, webbed neck, low hairline) and amenorrhea. However, women with genetic mosaicism in which only a portion of all cells have the 45,X karyotype may have normal phenotypes with regular menses during their early reproductive years. Their fertility may also be normal, but their inherent supply of oocytes is still compromised, leading to early ovarian failure. Some women may have short arm deletions of the X chromosome that lead to only partial expression of a Turner syndrome phenotype but still lead to early ovarian failure. Others may have abnormal karyotypes that include portions of a Y chromosome, putting them in a high risk category for gonadal tumors (e.g., dysgerminoma). These women should undergo bilateral oophorectomy as soon as their abnormal karyotype is discovered in order to mitigate their risk. For this reason, all women who experience ovarian failure prior to age 30 should have a karyotype performed.

Table 8.4 Etiologies of premature ovarian failure

Turner syndrome (± mosaicism)
Partial deletions of the X chromosome
Fragile X syndrome premutation
Somatic chromosomal defects*
Chemotherapy
Radiation therapy
Ovarian surgery including oophorectomy
Viral infection
Autoimmune ovarian failure
Polyglandular autoimmune syndromes I and II
Galactosemia*
Steroidogenic enzyme deficiencies*
Luteinizing hormone and follicle-stimulating hormone receptor mutations*
Idiopathic

*Associated with premature ovarian failure and primary amenorrhea.

Fragile X syndrome is an X-linked form of mental retardation that is the most common cause of mental retardation in males worldwide. Women who carry premutations in the *FMR1* gene that causes fragile X syndrome have a 16% risk for premature ovarian failure. Although women with premature ovarian failure are unlikely to have more children once their diagnosis has been made, their offspring and siblings may still be planning to have children, in which case proper screening for *FMR1* premutations may help them better understand their risk of this potentially devastating condition.

Premature ovarian failure may also occur as a result of autoimmune processes that can affect multiple organ systems. The most common autoimmune disease associated with it is Hashimoto thyroiditis, necessitating the need for early screening and surveillance of TSH and antithyroid peroxidase and antithyroglobulin antibodies. Other autoimmune diseases such as diabetes and adrenal failure are much less common but are potentially devastating sequelae of ongoing illness. As a result, assessment of fasting glucose and insulin along with measurement of serum antiadrenal and anti-21-hydroxylase antibodies is warranted at the time of diagnosis and yearly thereafter. If antiadrenal antibodies are found, referral for an adrenocorticotropin (ACTH; Cortrosyn) stimulation test is warranted to indicate whether adrenal insufficiency might result in times of severe stress. In the case of insufficient adrenal responsiveness to ACTH stimulation, a MedicAlert bracelet should be worn by the patient, and injectable cortisone should be readily available in the case of an emergency. Past recommendations for testing for antiovarian antibodies and ovarian biopsy are no longer indicated because of their poor sensitivity and predictive value.

Anatomic causes of amenorrhea

Genital tract abnormalities are found in the setting of normal hormonal parameters with a failed response to a progestin challenge. Congenital anomalies of the female genital tract are associated with primary amenorrhea rather than secondary amenorrhea, and include müllerian agenesis (Mayer–Rokitansky–Kuster–Hauser syndrome) and androgen insensitivity. Müllerian agenesis is characterized by a short, blind-ending vagina with rudimentary uterine anlagen, usually attached by a fibrous band in the midline. Ovaries and tubes are normal, but there may be associated renal, vertebral, and, less often, auditory and cardiac defects. Androgen insensitivity is also associated with a short, blind-ending vagina, but no müllerian structures develop and gonads are true testes that are often found in the inguinal canals. Patients with müllerian agenesis are phenotypically normal, whereas those with androgen insensitivity have a female phenotype and are typically tall and thin with scant pubic and axillary hair. The two may be differentiated by a serum testosterone level, which should be in the normal male range for androgen insensitivity patients. A 46,XY karyotype provides a definitive diagnosis of androgen insensitivity.

Other anatomic defects that may present with amenorrhea include cervical agenesis, transverse vaginal septum, and imperforate hymen. These conditions usually present with cyclic pain due to accumulation of blood behind the obstruction. Occasionally, an intact hymen may have microperforations that allow a limited amount of flow with every menses. Diagnostic evaluation of lower genital tract obstruction requires imaging with transperineal ultrasound, MRI, or both. If an imperforate hymen or transverse vaginal septum is suspected, one should never attempt to insert a needle through it to aspirate vaginal contents because of potential bacterial seeding and ascending infection. After a definitive diagnosis has been made with imaging studies, surgical repair should be accomplished by a gynecologic surgeon familiar with such procedures. In the case of cervical agenesis, most patients are best treated with hysterectomy because of only a minimal degree of success in creating patent outflow tracts using various techniques. Instances of pregnancy following transmyometrial embryo transfer have, however, been reported in such cases.

> ### ✋ CAUTION!
>
> Never attempt to insert a needle through a suspected hymen because of potential bacterial seeding and resultant fulminant infection.

The most common condition of the genital tract leading to secondary amenorrhea is the presence of intrauterine adhesions or syechiae, also known as Asherman syndrome. The typical scenario leading to the development of adhesions involves curettage for pregnancy complications such as incomplete abortion, postpartum hemorrhage, or retained placental fragments. Concomitant infection further increases the risk for adhesions. In the developing world, genital tuberculosis still accounts for a large number of cases in which the endometrial cavity may be completely obliterated. Treatment is surgical using hysteroscopic techniques that include lysis of adhesions with small scissors, or electrocautery under laparoscopic or ultrasound guidance. Reformation of adhesions is a major concern following these procedures, prompting many surgeons to use intrauterine balloons or stents with supplemental estrogen postoperatively as preventive measures. Data regarding the efficacy of such measures are lacking, however.

Severe cervical stenosis can also lead to secondary amenorrhea or scant menstrual flow and should be a consideration for possible outflow obstruction. Most cases arise after some type of cervical procedure such as LEEP or cryotherapy for treatment of cervical intraepithelial neoplasia. Risk of stenosis after these procedures is heightened when infection is present, emphasizing the need for antibiotic prophylaxis in high-risk individuals. Other less common causes of stenosis or obstruction during the reproductive years include cervical fibroids and cancer.

If an atypical lesion like these is present, office biopsy is necessary to direct appropriate treatment. For most cases, however, serial dilatation in the office after appropriate application of a cervical block with 1% lidocaine is indicated. Severe cases may require use of extremely small wire dilators or lacrimal duct probes, with or without simultaneous transabdominal ultrasound guidance. Pretreatment of a stenotic cervix with vaginal misoprostol 400 µg the night before attempted dilatation can soften the consistency of the cervix and facilitate dilator insertion. Patients should be cautioned regarding the possibility of stomach upset, cramping, and diarrhea with misoprostol, while healthcare providers should screen for pregnancy before prescribing the drug due to its abortifacient property.

> ☆ **TIPS & TRICKS**
>
> Before attempting to dilate a stenotic cervix, have the patient insert 400 µg of misoprostol vaginally the night before her office visit to soften the cervix.

Summary

Particular causes of amenorrhea may represent life-threatening clinical conditions. Historical information and appropriate testing are critical to guide the clinician toward a prompt and specific diagnosis for these women. A different profile of clinical disorders will be found when evaluating women with primary versus secondary amenorrhea.

Selected bibliography

American Psychiatric Association. Diagnostic and statistical manual of mental disorders, 4th ed. Washington, DC: American Psychiatric Association, 1994.

Domar AD, Clapp D, Slawsby E, Kessel B, Orav J, Freizinger M. The impact of group psychological interventions on distress in infertile women. Health Psychol 2000;19: 568–76.

March WA, Moore VM, Willson KJ, Phillips DI, Norman RJ, Davies MJ. The prevalence of polycystic ovary syndrome in a community sample assessed under contrasting diagnostic criteria. Hum Reprod 2010;25:544–51.

)Molitch ME. Pathologic hyperprolactinemia. Endocrinol Metab Clin North Am 1992;21: 877–901.

Pettersson F, Fries H, Nillius SJ. Epidemiology of secondary amenorrhea: incidence and prevalence rates. Am J Obstet Gynecol 1973;117:80–6.

Reindollar RH, Novak M, Tho SP, McDonough PG. Adult-onset amenorrhea: a study of 262 patients. Am J Obstet Gynecol 1986;155: 531–43.

Schlechte J, Sherman B, Halmi N et al. Prolactin-secreting pituitary tumors in amenorrheic women: a comprehensive study. Endocr Rev 1980;1:295–308.

Schlechte JA, Sherman BM, Chapler FK, Van Gilder J. Long term follow-up of women with surgically treated prolactin-secreting pituitary tumors. J Clin Endocrinol Metab 1986;62:1296–301.

9

Menstrual Cycle-related Clinical Disorders

Paul B. Marshburn

Carolinas Medical Center, Charlotte, North Carolina, USA

Premenstrual syndrome

Premenstrual syndrome (PMS) refers to the cyclic appearance of distressing symptoms just prior to the menses that significantly impairs social, physical, or occupational functioning. These symptoms are distressing for approximately 20% of reproductive-aged women, and about 5% have premenstrual symptoms severe enough to disrupt the performance of social or work activities. The average age at onset of PMS is around 26 years, yet the condition can gradually worsens over time until menopause. Without relief of symptoms, a woman who develops the disorder at age 26 may experience an average of 2,800 symptomatic days before she reaches menopause. Studies indicate that the degree of impairment in social and leisure activities, marital relationships, parental activities, and extended family activities is similar to that associated with major depressive disorder.

The symptoms of PMS are characterized by dysfunctional mood, often with physical and behavioral changes that occur during the late luteal phase of a woman's menstrual cycle. These impairing symptoms are relieved soon after the onset of menses. Diagnostic criteria for PMS have been defined by the American College of Obstetricians and Gynecologists (ACOG). The ACOG Practice Bulletin defines PMS as the presence of at least one affective (depression, angry outbursts, irritability, anxiety, confusion, social withdrawal) and somatic (breast tenderness, abdominal bloating, headache, swelling of extremities) symptom during the 5 days before menses in each of three prospectively charted cycles. The American Psychiatric Association has established diagnostic criteria for premenstrual dysphoric disorder (PMDD) that include irritability, anger, mood swings, depression, tension/anxiety, abdominal bloating, breast pain and fatigue. In this chapter, PMS and PMDD will be used interchangeably because the treatment strategies are the same. A diagnosis of PMDD is reserved for women who meet the *Diagnostic and Statistical Manual of Mental Disorders* criteria of at least 5 of 11 total symptoms, one of which must be a core symptom (depressed mood, anxiety or tension, affective lability, or irritability). The diagnosis of PMS/PMDD is made only after exclusion of signs or symptoms that are caused by other primary medical or psychiatric disorders. Historical inquiry, a thorough physical examination, and laboratory testing should seek to determine whether other medical or psychiatric disorders are present (Table 9.1).

At the initial consultation, the effective physician needs to establish a trusting relationship with the patient by reassurance that her distressing symptoms can be explained by a defined clinical disorder. The patient is often relieved that further evaluation will be undertaken to evaluate the possibility that other medical or psychiatric

Disorders of Menstruation, 1st edition. Edited by Paul B. Marshburn and Bradley S. Hurst.
© 2011 Blackwell Publishing Ltd.

Table 9.1 Common conditions in the differential diagnosis of premenstrual syndrome/premenstrual dysphoric disorder

Psychiatric disorders	Medical disorders	Premenstrual exacerbation	Psychosocial issues
Anorexia or bulimia	Allergies	Anemia	Sexual abuse
Bipolar disorder	Anemia	Cancer	Domestic violence
Dysthymia	Autoimmune disorders	Endocrine disorders	
Generalized anxiety	Seizure disorder	Endometriosis	
Major depression	Perimenopause	Lupus erythematosus	
Panic disorder	Collagen vascular disease	Seizure disorder	
Personality disorder	Diabetes mellitus		
Somatoform disorder	Dysmenorrhea		
Substance abuse	Endometriosis Hypothyroidism Migraine Oral contraceptive pill use Chronic fatigue syndrome		

Reproduced from Jarvis et al., 2008, with permission.

disorders are the root cause of the problem. While some of the clinical entities listed in the differential diagnosis may worsen in the premenstrual phase, they are not considered PMS/PMDD but rather symptoms associated with that medical or psychiatric disorder. Specific treatment to address these other primary medical or psychiatric disorders will often eliminate debilitating premenstrual symptoms.

The diagnosis of PMS/PMDD requires 3 months of prospective symptom ratings, which can be accomplished utilizing a validated calendar charting such as the Calendar of Premenstrual Experiences [COPE] (Figure 9.1). To arrive at a diagnosis of PMS/PMDD, the calendar should reveal at least a twofold increase in total symptom severity during the last week prior to the initiation of menses compared with the second week of the cycle, counting day 1 as the first day of menses. It should be explained to patients that if the diagnosis of PMS/PMDD is indicated by prospective symptom charting, therapy with proven efficacy will be provided.

Prior to the initiation of prospective symptom charting, the physician should educate the patient that healthy lifestyle choices can improve distressing premenstrual symptoms. Instruct the patient to include aerobic exercise, good sleep hygiene, and caffeine and tobacco limitation during the 2-month charting period. Improvement in PMS symptoms can also be achieved with over-the-counter vitamins and minerals. Vitamin B_6 (50 mg per day), magnesium (375 mg per day), and calcium (1200 mg per day) therapy produced modest relief from PMS symptoms in prospective, controlled trials. Investigate the home atmosphere to assess the potential for familial discord or abuse, and enlist the support of a caring partner to help the vulnerable patient. Any changes that allow patients to exert greater control over their lives will produce a favorable impact. In this manner, the patient can initiate healthy measures that impart the sense that therapy has begun. A patient may return after charting with a significant improvement in symptoms, significantly aided by a desire to please the caring physician.

Name _____ Month/Year _____ Age _____ Unit# _____

Begin your calendar on the first day of your menstrual cycle. Enter the calendar date below the cycle day.
Day 1 is your first day of bleeding.
Shade the box above the cycle day if you have bleeding ▨
Put an X for spotting ☒
If more than one symptom is listed in a category, ie, nausea, diarrhea, constipation, you do not need to experience all of these. Rate the most disturbing of the symptoms on the 1–3 scale.

Weight: weigh yourself before breakfast. Record weight in the box below date.
Symptoms: Indicate the severity of your symptoms by using the scale below.
Rate each symptom at about the same time each evening.
0: None present (symptom not present) 1: Mild (noticeable but not troublesome)
2: Moderate (interferes with normal activities) 3: Severe (intolerable, unable to perform normal activities)
Other Symptoms: If there are other symptoms you experience, list and indicate severity.
Medications: List any medications taken. Put an X on the corresponding day(s).

Bleeding																														
Cycle day	1	2	3	4	5	6	7	8	9	10	11	12	13	14	15	16	17	18	19	20	21	22	23	24	25	26	27	28	29	30
Date																														
Weight																														
Symptoms																														
Acne																														
Bloatedness																														
Breast tenderness																														
Dizziness																														
Fatigue																														
Headache																														
Hot flashes																														
Nausea, diarrhea, constipation																														
Palpitations																														
Swelling (hands, ankles, breast)																														
Angry outbursts, arguments, violent tendencies																														
Anxiety, tension, nervousness																														
Confusion, difficulty concentrating																														
Crying easily																														
Depression																														
Food cravings (sweets, salts)																														
Forgetfulness																														
Irritability																														
Increased appetite																														
Mood swings																														
Overly sensitive																														
Wish to be alone																														
Other symptoms 1. 2.																														
Medications 1. 2.																														

Figure 9.1 Calendar of Premenstrual Experiences for the diagnosis of premenstrual syndrome. Reproduced from Mortola et al. 1990 © University of California, San Diego: Department of Reproductive Medicine, H:813; Division of Reproductive Endocrinology.

★ TIPS AND TRICKS

In managing premenstrual syndrome, avoid proceeding with prospective symptom charting without first: (1) reassuring the patient that her symptoms have a clinical basis; (2) instituting lifestyle changes that may help premenstrual syndrome symptoms; and (3) initiating diagnostic evaluation to rule out other potential medical disorders. This practice will engender a trusting relationship and knowledge that therapy has begun.

If prospective charting indicates the diagnosis of PMS/PMDD, steps should be taken to analyze whether symptoms can be grouped under a categorical heading. Such principal categories include: affective symptoms (depression, irritability, lack of pleasure and interest in life's activities, mood lability, anxiety), fluid retention (mastalgia, bloating, headache), and menstrual pain (dysmenorrhea). Most cases of PMS will have affective symptoms that dominate the symptom complex.

Targeting therapy towards a symptom category can allow tailoring of treatment to the woman's principal complaints (Table 9.2). Relief of fluid retention symptoms may be relieved by low doses of spironolactone (50 mg twice daily). If spironolactone is prescribed, reliable contraception is needed (as it is a Food and Drug Administration [FDA] Pregnancy Category D drug), and periodic serum potassium monitoring is necessary. A dopamine agonist such as bromocriptine or cabergoline is most efficacious for isolated mastalgia. Physical symptoms associated with menstrual pain may be relieved by premenstrual nonsteroidal anti-inflammatory drugs (NSAIDs) and oral contraceptive medication (especially a combined oral contraceptive pill [OCP] with drospirenone as its progestin). OCPs with drospirenone have FDA approval for management of PMDD. The suppression of ovulation with OCPs may improve a broad range of mood and behavioral disturbances in addition to physical premenstrual symptoms.

The efficacy of selective serotonin reuptake inhibitors (SSRIs) for the affective symptoms of PMS/PMDD is well established. Fluoxetine, controlled-release paroxetine, and sertraline are the only FDA-approved SSRI agents for the treatment of PMS/PMDD. A dosing regimen of SSRIs during the luteal phase only was found to be slightly less effective than a continuous dosing regimen. Physician familiarity with the adverse effects of SSRIs is important so that pretreatment counseling can be given. In particular, sexual side effects following SSRI treatment, such as reduced libido and anorgasmia, have been reported. Strategies to diminish these sexual side effects include decreasing the dose, switching to another SSRI, or taking drug holidays. Switching from a continuous to a luteal phase-only dosing regimen would be an alternative method to minimize these sexual side effects.

The administration of SSRIs in addition to other serotonergic agonists (e.g., triptans for migraine headache) should be avoided to limit the serious consequences of the "serotonin syndrome."

⚠ CAUTION!

Serotonin syndrome is a potentially life-threatening condition associated with inadvertent interactions between drugs that enhance serotonergic activity. *For this reason, coadministration of selective serotonin reuptake inhibitors and triptans, used for migraine treatment (see below), should be avoided.* Serotonin syndrome is characterized by a triad of mental status changes (anxiety, agitated delirium, restlessness, disorientation), autonomic hyperactivity (diaphoresis, tachycardia, hyperthermia, hypertension, vomiting, diarrhea), and neuromuscular abnormalities (tremor, muscle rigidity, myoclonus, hyperreflexia). Treatment involves discontinuation of all serotonergic agents, supportive care aimed at normalization of vital signs, sedation with benzodiazepines, and in severe cases administration of serotonin antagonists (cyproheptadine). Intensive care unit support may be necessary.

Table 9.2 Prescription medications recommended for use in the treatment of premenstrual syndrome (PMS)/premenstrual dysphoric disorder

Drug class and agents	Dosage	Recommendations for use	Adverse effects
Affective symptoms			
Fluoxetine	10–20 mg/day (max 60 mg/day)	First-line for somatic and mood symptoms (intermittent therapy)	Sexual dysfunction, sleep disturbances (sedation, hypersomnia), gastrointestinal distress, fatigue, headache, nervousness
Sertraline	50–150 mg/day		
Paroxetine controlled release	20–30 mg/day		
Anxiolytics			
Alprazolam	0.75–1.0 mg/day (max 4.0 mg/day)	Second-line for anxiety (intermittent therapy)	Drowsiness, sedation, risk of dependence, tolerance development
Menstrual pain			
Nonsteroidal anti-inflammatory drugs		Effective in alleviating physical symptoms of PMS	Nausea, gastric ulceration, renal dysfunction
Naproxen sodium	275–550 mg twice daily as needed up to 1–2 days before cramps or menstrual cycle begins, until symptoms resolve		
Ethinylestradiol/drospirenone-containing oral contraceptive pills	Yaz: 20 μg ethinylestradiol/3 mg drospirenone daily for 24 days	Effective in alleviating some PMS symptoms; symptoms may worsen in some women	Breast tenderness, nausea, irregular bleeding, thrombosis, hyperkalemia
Gonadotropin-releasing hormone agonists		Effective for psychoemotional and physical symptoms	Hypoestrogenic adverse effects including atrophic vaginitis, hot flashes, and osteoporosis
Leuprolide	3.75 mg intramuscularly every month or 11.25 mg intramuscularly every 3 months	Adverse effect profile and cost limit use, especially long term (>6 months) "Add-back" therapy with estrogen and/or progesterone if used >6 months	
Fluid retention			
Spironolactone	25–200 mg/day during luteal phase	Effective in alleviating breast tenderness and bloating	Antiestrogen effects, hyperkalemia

If patients are refractory to first-line pharmaco-therapy for PMS/PDDD, gonadotropin-releasing hormone (GnRH) agonists are an effective alternative treatment. GnRH agonist administration is more efficacious for physical than behavioral symptoms. Hormonal add-back therapy (in typical continuous postmenopausal hormone doses) will reduce hypoestrogenic side effects but will not compromise efficacy. Approximately 60–70% of refractory patients will have a favorable response to GnRH agonist therapy.

An algorithm for management of PMS is presented here (Figure 9.2). Further clinically relevant research and assessments are still needed to optimize care for women who suffer from this disorder.

Dysmenorrhea

Dysmenorrhea is the occurrence of painful uterine cramps during the menses. This common gynecologic complaint may begin with the initiation of menses at puberty or develop secondarily during the reproductive years. Primary dysmen-

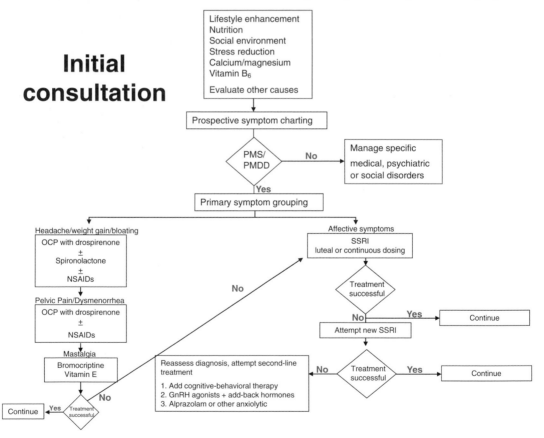

Figure 9.2 Algorithm for the management of premenstrual syndrome (PMS)/premenstrual dysphoric disorder (PMDD). GnRH, gonadotropin-releasing hormone; NSAID, nonsteroidal anti-inflammatory drug; OCP, oral contraceptive pill; SSRI, selective serotonin reuptake inhibitor.

orrhea is more prevalent in mid- and late adolescence when ovulation becomes more frequent. The premenstrual decline of progesterone and estrogen that occurs if pregnancy is not established produces higher levels of endometrial and uterine prostaglandins, hormones known to cause crampy abdominal menstrual pain. The negative effect on a sufferer's quality of life may be profound with incapacitating pain. Furthermore, dysmenorrhea may herald the existence of other conditions requiring alternative therapeutic approaches.

The differential diagnosis that should be considered with a history of dysmenorrhea includes obstructive müllerian anomalies, endometriosis, ectopic or failed intrauterine pregnancy, primary bowel disease, submucosal uterine neoplasms, and less commonly pelvic inflammatory disease. If a history, careful physical examination, and judicious laboratory testing (including pregnancy testing) do not suggest a cause for the dysmenorrhea, pelvic imaging with ultrasound or magnetic resonance imaging is warranted. Initial medical management for dysmenorrhea (described below) is appropriate if no other cause(s) of painful menses are discovered.

Approximately 60% of adolescent women who do not respond to pharmacologic treatment will have pelvic endometriosis discovered at laparoscopy. These young women often report progressive dysmenorrhea along with *acyclic pelvic pain* in 63% of cases. The endometriosis lesions discovered at the time of laparoscopy in adolescents are more commonly "clear" or "red" vesicular lesions rather than the classic "powder burn" lesions seen in more mature reproductive-aged women (Figure 9.3). The finding of continuous pelvic pain in adolescent women in association with endometriosis contrasts with the more common endometriosis presentation of solitary progressive dysmenorrhea in older reproductive-age women.

The most common medical therapies for dysmenorrhea are combined oral contraceptive pills and nonsteroidal anti-inflammatory drugs. Both agents act by suppressing endometrial and uterine prostaglandin levels.

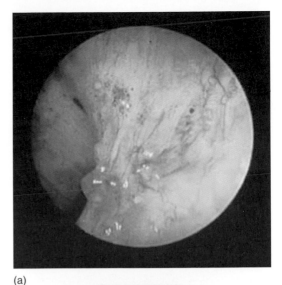

(a)

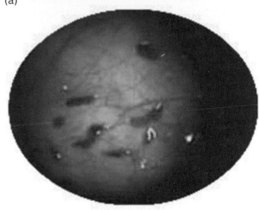

(b)

Figure 9.3 Appearance of (a) clear and (b) red endometriosis lesions seen in adolescents (see Plate 9.3).

Nonsteroidal anti-inflammatory agents act to reduce pain-causing prostaglandins by directly inhibiting prostaglandin synthesis. Oral contraceptives act indirectly by inhibiting ovulation and by progestin-induced thinning of the endometrial lining, which will reduce menstrual fluid volume and prostaglandin levels.

Clinical trials document that NSAIDs are an effective treatment for dysmenorrhea. There is insufficient evidence to indicate any particular NSAID that is the safest and most effective for dysmenorrhea treatment. Women using NSAIDs

Table 9.3 Nonsteroidal anti-inflammatory drugs for the treatment of primary dysmenorrhea

Drug	Dosage
Ibuprofen	200–600 mg every 6 hours as needed
Naproxen sodium	440–550 mg initially, with 220–275 mg every 8 hours as needed
Mefenamic acid	500 mg initially, with 250 mg every 6 hours as needed
Celecoxib[a,b]	400 mg initially, with 200 mg every 12 hours as needed

[a] For girls over 18 years.
[b] Cyclooxygenase-2 specific inhibitor.

need to be aware of the potential adverse effect of gastrointestinal upset, headaches, and occasionally drowsiness. A loading dose of NSAIDs may be given initially, and the medication should be started prior to the onset of menses (Table 9.3).

The use of combined OCPs is effective treatment for primary dysmenorrhea. Several small, randomized controlled trials have found that combined OCPs with medium-dose estrogen (35 µg) and first-/second-generation progestins (such as norethindrone and levonorgestrel) were more effective than placebo for menstrual cramps associated with dysmenorrhea. Lower-dose combined OCPs have less evidence to support their efficacy in treating dysmenorrhea, although improved outcomes for days missed from work or school have been observed following low-dose OCP treatment. In clinical trials, no difference was found in the occurrence of adverse effects between OCPs and placebo. The use of a continuous regimen of OCPs would logically be assumed to be superior to cyclic OCP administration in the management of dysmenorrhea, but there are insufficient data to document the merits of continuous OCPs in the treatment of dysmenorrhea.

Approximately 20–25% of women who suffer from dysmenorrhea will fail to have relief from NSAID and/or OCP treatment. Although behavioral approaches such as cognitive therapy may have slight therapeutic benefit, results from small poorly controlled studies are inconclusive. Laparoscopic uterine nerve ablation procedures (performed by transection of the uterosacral ligaments) have produced no long-term benefit in recalcitrant dysmenorrhea. Presacral neurectomy surgery, however, is effective in the management of central pelvic pain and dysmenorrhea in patients with endometriosis.

Systematic reviews of other therapies for dysmenorrhea have been published in the Cochrane Database. The progestin-containing intrauterine device, endometrial ablation, and hysterectomy have all been effectively employed to manage dysmenorrhea refractory to systemic medical therapy. Small studies suggest a potential benefit with the use of Chinese herbal medicine for primary dysmenorrhea; however, the poor quality of available trials limits conclusions about treatment efficacy. No evidence was found to recommend spinal manipulation therapy, transcutaneous electrical nerve stimulation, acupuncture, or vitamin B_1 and magnesium treatment for therapy to relieve dysmenorrhea.

Menstrual migraines

Migraine headaches are three times more common in women. Cyclic changes in estradiol and progesterone during the menstrual cycle modulate central neuronal activity and may cause a change in the incidence and intensity of headache. A trigger for menstrual cycle-associated migraine headache is thought to be a significant drop in blood estrogen levels that occurs during the 2–3 days prior to onset of menses. This hormonal mechanism is supported by the observation that the frequency of migraines in women increases considerably after menarche and during the perimenopausal transition. Pure menstrual migraine (MM) is a headache event that occurs exclusively at the time of menses (8–14% of all women migraineurs), while 60% of women may simply experience an increased migraine severity or frequency at menstruation (menstrually related migraine). Women presenting with recurrent migraine headache require a complete diagnostic evaluation to fully assess the presence of other headache disorders and other intracranial abnormalities. Consultation with neurologists who specialize in headache management is recommended to direct an optimal therapeutic approach.

Migraine headache is lateralized in 60% of cases, and is often preceded by premonitory symptoms (fatigue, nausea, sensitivity to light) for several hours or longer. Aura is a complex of neurologic symptoms (visual, sensory, motor, or speech disturbances) that may accompany migraines and typically precedes the onset of the headache. A prospective headache diary is essential in determining the timing of headache symptoms and their relationship to precipitating factors. Precipitating and exacerbating factors (besides estrogen withdrawal) include stress, worry, exertion, fatigue, lack of sleep, not eating, and certain foods containing nitrites, glutamate, aspartate, and tyramine. MM is usually not associated with aura even in women who have migraine with aura at other times. There is some evidence that MM attacks are longer, more severe, and more resistant to treatment than other migraines.

Patient diaries that record headache onset, relationship to the menstrual cycle events, and response to treatment will suggest MM. Because most MM attacks occur after ovulatory cycles, the predictability of menses permits a tailored use of prophylactic medications. The initial *acute* treatment of MM is the same as migraines that occur at other times. Triptan medications have been shown to be effective in relieving MM. If aura is present, triptans should be administered when the aura is over and the headache pain is beginning. Effective acute treatment of MM includes the administration of sumatriptan 50–100 mg or rizatriptan 10 mg. Combination therapy of a triptan with an NSAID (such as mefenamic acid) is an option for women with both headache and menstrual symptoms.

Some patients may require *preventative* therapy for MM based on suboptimal response to an adequate trial of acute therapy. Preventative therapies for MM can be either nonspecific (those which do not address the hormonal trigger) or specific (hormonal strategies). Triptan

treatment 2 days before anticipated menses and continued for 5 days has shown an up to 50% reduction in the number of headache events and their severity (sumatriptan 25 mg three times per day, naratriptan 1 mg twice daily, frovatriptan 2.5 mg twice daily). One study indicated modest preventative benefit from naproxen sodium (550 mg twice daily) beginning 7 days before expected menses and continued for 13 days.

✋ CAUTION!

This benefit of naproxen sodium in the management of menstrual migraine should be balanced against the Food and Drug Administration warning of potential cardiovascular adverse events with the administration of naproxen sodium at higher doses. Current dosage recommendations for naproxen sodium are to not exceed 220 mg twice daily and for no longer than 10 days unless a physician directs otherwise. Oral contraceptive pills should *not* be administered to women who have migraine headache with aura at any time.

Hormonal prophylactic strategies that offset the premenstrual decline in estradiol may be effective for MM in women who do not respond to nonspecific treatment strategies. Continuous OCP administration for extended periods of time will suppress ovulation and menses. In the case of MM *without aura*, these cyclic headaches can be avoided for months at a time by the administration of continuous OCPs. The use of combined OCPs in women who have migraine headache *with aura* should be avoided. ACOG has concluded that the risks of OCPs outweigh the benefits in women over age 35 whose migraines are complicated by focal neurologic deficits. In women who have migraine *without aura* at all times, an extended-cycle OCP regimen may provide effective prevention. When using extended-cycle regimens that allow for periodic menses, estrogen supplementation is recommended during the placebo week. A 0.1 mg per day estradiol patch may be started 2 days before the placebo pills and will usually prevent MM.

Some women who have contraindications to the use of oral contraceptives may still be candidates for targeted strategies using low-dose estrogen, such as the perimenstrual transcutaneous administration of estradiol (0.1 mg per day patch). Orally administered sublingual micronized estradiol (1 mg) has also been effective if given 48 hours prior to the anticipated onset of menstrual migraines and continued for 6 days. Estrogen supplementation should *not* be started prior to 6 days before the first full day of menstruation, with continuation into the first 2 days of menses, because rebound migraine may occur after the estrogen supplement is stopped.

GnRH agonists such as leuprolide acetate can markedly diminish MM. This salutary effect of GnRH agonists is not compromised by continuous estrogen and progestin add-back therapy at postmenopausal doses. GnRH agonists are not approved by the FDA for the management of MM. For this reason, the expense, and the hypoestrogenic side effects, GnRH agonist treatment for MM should be a last resort.

In summary, the initial treatment of MM should be the same as for migraine occurring at any time: a triptan administered early in the mild pain stage. If this strategy does not provide relief, preventative therapy with triptans, extended-cycle combined hormonal contraceptives, regular-cycle OCPs with supplemental estrogen, or targeted supplemental estrogen may be indicated. Nonhormonal options are necessary for women who have contraindications to estrogen and progestin use (such as MM with aura). The gynecologic physician should develop familiarity with the precautions and side effects of a given triptan medication, and should avoid prescribing triptans if other medications that interact with the serotonergic system (such as SSRIs) are needed (see the Caution box above about serotonin syndrome). An initial consultation with a neurologist specializing in migraine headache is recommended for the management of patients with MM.

Catamenial epilepsy

Catamenial epilepsy is a menstrual cycle-related seizure disorder that affects up to 70% of women with epilepsy. These women suffer increased seizure frequency during the time near ovulation and in the premenstrual phase, a time when the ratio of serum estrogen (proconvulsant) to serum progesterone (anticonvulsant) is high. An increase in frequency of seizures has also been demonstrated during anovulatory cycles when progesterone levels are relatively low.

Animal studies indicate that estrogen dominance may increase seizure susceptibility by: (1) activating central excitatory glutamate neurotransmission, while (2) suppressing the inhibitory neurotransmission of gamma-aminobutyric acid (GABA) neurons. Conversely, progesterone may reduce seizure susceptibility partly through conversion to neuronally active steroids, such as allopregnanolone, which enhances GABA(A) receptor function and thereby inhibits neuronal excitability.

Women with epilepsy are more likely to have reproductive disorders such as polycystic ovarian syndrome (PCOS), early menopause, and anovulatory menstrual cycles than are women in the general population. Increasing evidence implicates both epilepsy itself and the antiepileptic drug (AED) valproic acid (Valproate) as contributing factors in reproductive disorders in women with epilepsy.

Neurologists who work in epilepsy consider catamenial seizures a challenge to manage with antiepileptic medication. Often a patient's seizures are well controlled except during the premenstrual phase. Increasing doses of antiepileptic medication premenstrually may be beneficial, but not all AED medications can be acutely increased before menses to significantly change blood levels. Furthermore, catamenial seizures may be attributed to changes in the metabolic clearance of anticonvulsant medication. Decreased levels of phenytoin have been demonstrated during menses in women with catamenial epilepsy, and this decrease correlates with increased seizure activity. The decrease in estrogen and progesterone at menstruation stimulates the release of hepatic monoxygenase enzymes, which accelerates anticonvulsant metabolism and increases the risk for breakthrough seizures. Treatment of catamenial epilepsy may require measurement of serum levels of anticonvulsants during times of seizure exacerbation, with attempts at altered dosing as appropriate to improve seizure control.

At present, there is no FDA-approved therapy for catamenial epilepsy, and existing pharmacotherapy for this disorder is largely empirical. The efficacy of treatments for catamenial seizures has been demonstrated from small, unblinded studies or anecdotal reports. A variety of therapies for catamenial seizures has been proposed, including targeted increases in conventional AEDs, acetazolamide administration, and hormonal therapy. A study of 20 women with catamenial seizures indicated that acetazolamide reduced seizure frequency by 40% and severity by 30%.

The role of progesterone as an anticonvulsant in catamenial seizures has emerged. Progestin treatment at times of increased seizure vulnerability (i.e., low circulating progesterone levels) would be predicted to have a beneficial therapeutic impact. Approximately 65% of the women who achieved progestin-induced amenorrhea experienced a mean reduction in seizure frequency of 30%. Not all synthetic progestins, however, are efficacious in the treatment of catamenial epilepsy. Norethisterone treatment has been shown to be ineffective in the control of catamenial seizures.

Orally administered micronized progesterone, at doses of 100–200 mg three times daily on days 15–28 of the menstrual cycle, reduced seizure frequency by about 60% during 3 years of treatment. This treatment was associated with increased fatigue, sedation, and mild depressive symptoms, but these adverse effects promptly resolved with a dose reduction. Depot medroxyprogesterone acetate (DMPA), 150 mg intramuscularly every 2 months, can decrease catamenial seizure activity by 50%. Long-term treatment with DMPA should be considered carefully because of the potential for osteoporosis with DMPA-induced amenorrhea. Medroxyprogesterone acetate proved effective in a small series of women with temporal lobe epilepsy.

> **⚠ CAUTION!**
>
> *Petit mal seizures have been reported to worsen with progestin administration.* Prior to progestin administration, discussion with the consulting neurologist should occur to establish the seizure type and the timing of seizure occurrence. Plans can be made with the consulting neurologist for the monitoring of serum antiepileptic drug levels during menses so that the antiepileptic drug dosage may be appropriately adjusted if necessary.

Animal studies provide data suggesting that the provision of stable hormonal levels with continuous OCPs may be effective. Limited clinical data indicate that continuous OCP treatment may provide impressive relief, but such treatment is not consistently effective. With OCP use, care must be taken because enzyme-inducing anticonvulsants may reduce plasma hormone levels. For this reason, the contraceptive efficacy of OCPs may be decreased in patients with epilepsy receiving anticonvulsant therapy. Thus a higher-dose (50 µg ethinylestradiol) OCP is recommended for contraceptive efficacy in women taking certain AEDs. Other ovarian suppressive agents, including danazol and GnRH agonist therapy with add-back, have not been sufficiently tested for controlling catamenial seizure. Controlled trials to evaluate the underlying pathophysiology of catamenial seizures, as well as its treatment options, are needed.

Women with epilepsy are more likely to have menstrual disorders than women in the general population. It is estimated that women with epilepsy have a twofold increase in oligo-ovulation compared to the general population. This association with anovulatory cycles may increase the risks for infertility, migraine, and endometrial cancer. Among the AEDs, valproate has been associated with the development of characteristic PCOS features. The risk appears to be particularly high when valproate use is started in childhood or adolescence. Menopause tends to occur earlier in women with epilepsy. The intricate relationship between reproductive disorders and epilepsy suggests that reproductive function should be monitored closely as part of the comprehensive care of women with epilepsy. Therefore, regular monitoring of reproductive function at visits, including questioning about menstrual disorders, fertility, weight, hirsutism, and galactorrhea, is recommended.

Other diseases and menstrual disorders

Cyclic changes in the severity of symptoms related to other medical conditions have been observed in women. The disorders discussed below show exacerbation in relation to particular phases of the menstrual cycle. The etiology and mechanism of disease expression in these conditions are, however, incompletely understood.

Asthma

The observation that asthma is influenced by cyclic changes in sex steroids is supported by the fact that asthma is more common in young women after puberty. Approximately 30–40% of women with asthma have an increased severity and/or frequency of asthma attacks in the premenstrual phase. The abrupt drop in progesterone prior to menstruation is associated with an alteration in prostaglandin release, changes in the immune system, and a reduction in progesterone's relaxant effect on bronchial smooth muscle. This worsening of asthmatic symptoms in the premenstrual phase is associated with a decrease in peak expiratory flow rates and an increase in serious respiratory complications.

The strategy of therapeutic intervention during the late luteal phase has been useful in the management of premenstrual exacerbation of asthma. Targeted drug therapy during the premenstrual phase for these asthmatic attacks has yielded clinical benefit from the administration of leukotriene receptor antagonists and long-acting inhaled beta-2 agonists. Longer-term treatment with progesterone and GnRH agonists has been helpful in some cases of recalcitrant premenstrual asthma. Further randomized controlled trials are required before the optimal drug therapy for premenstrual asthma is established.

Rheumatoid arthritis

Symptoms of rheumatoid arthritis (RA) often improve in the luteal phase and during pregnancy, while morning stiffness and arthritic pain tend to worsen during menses and the postpartum period. These observations have led to the conclusion that times of high estrogen and progesterone levels are associated with a reduction in the symptoms of RA, although the mechanism of this effect is unknown. Combination OCPs have proven beneficial in RA by delaying the onset and severity of arthritic symptoms. OCPs, however, will not prevent the occurrence of RA. Postmenopausal estrogen and estrogen/progestin therapy does *not* appear to be effective in providing symptomatic relief from RA.

Irritable bowel syndrome

Irritable bowel syndrome (IBS) is characterized by chronic or recurrent abdominal pain, and altered bowel habits (diarrhea and constipation) with no evidence of structural, infectious, or other gastrointestinal disease process. Symptoms of IBS are much more common in women, and exacerbation of symptoms occurs commonly during the postovulatory and premenstrual phases of the menstrual cycle. Progesterone's effect to relax gastrointestinal smooth muscle and delay gastric emptying is associated with constipation in the luteal phase in IBS sufferers. Progesterone withdrawal with menses may trigger an increase in bowel activity with the appearance of diarrhea. Prostaglandin inhalers and GnRH agonists have demonstrated some benefit is small clinical studies. The common concurrence of IBS and endometriosis should be remembered in the management of these patients.

Diseases associated with menstrual irregularities

The association between insulin resistance and PCOS is well understood. The chronic oligomenorrhea associated with PCOS is often alleviated with the improved insulin sensitivity that follows weight loss or metformin treatment (see other chapters). Women with *type 1 diabetes* also have a higher incidence of menstrual irregularities (amenorrhea, oligomenorrhea). These menstrual abnormalities appear to be secondary to dysfunction of the hypothalamic GnRH pulse generator. Clinical observations demonstrate that diabetic ketoacidosis, severe insulin reactions, and hypoglycemic episodes worsen around the menses.

Psychotropic drug therapy for *schizophrenia* and *bipolar disorder* can disrupt the menstrual cycle, alter pregnancy potential, and increase the risk for chronic conditions such as PCOS. As discussed in the section on catamenial epilepsy, valproic acid has been associated with clinical features of PCOS. Certain antipsychotic medications used to treat schizophrenia (e.g., haloperidol, resperidol) act by dopamine receptor inhibition in the central nervous system. Dopamine receptor inhibition can increase prolactin production, which will disrupt cyclic gonadotropin (luteinizing hormone and follicle-stimulating hormone) release and ultimately lead to hypogonadotropic amenorrhea. The effects of dopamine receptor antagonists may reduce or prevent fertility and increase the risk for osteoporosis by lowering ovarian estradiol production. Counseling is required before initiating treatment in reproductive-age women who need these psychotropic medications.

Menstrual problems are common among women with *chronic kidney disease.* Patients with end-stage renal disease often exhibit amenorrhea, and fertility potential is reduced in patients with chronic kidney disease by about 50%. If pregnancy occurs, premature delivery is common. Consistent hemodialysis and kidney transplantation have greatly improved conception rates and pregnancy outcome in these women. Contraceptive counseling should be provided before transplantation, because ovulatory cycles may begin within 1–2 months after transplantation in women with functioning grafts.

Summary

The diagnosis of menstrual cycle-related clinical disorders requires the documentation of consistent cyclic symptoms with prospective reporting. The cyclic changes in estrogen and progesterone have a well-known physiologic and at times deleterious impact on genital and central nervous system function in women. Most of these disorders are associated with regular ovulatory cycles rather than abnormal reproductive cycles. This fact proves to be of great clinical advantage to the physician, because the application of therapy at a predictable phase of the menstrual cycle can help patients to benefit from preventative and targeted therapeutic intervention. Close collaboration with medical consultants will often provide the optimum outcome for patients. If targeted therapy is ineffectual, menstrual cycle-related disorders may be improved by a regimen of continuous, combination estrogen and progestin therapy, or GnRH agonist administration including estrogen plus progestin add-back therapy. Ovarian removal or ablation for recalcitrant and severe cases is very rarely employed in the modern management of these disorders.

Selected bibliography

Bauer J, Cooper-Mahkorn D. Reproductive dysfunction in women with epilepsy: menstrual cycle abnormalities, fertility, and polycystic ovary syndrome. Int Rev Neurobiol 2008;83:135–55.

Farage MA, Osborn TW, MacLean AB. Cognitive, sensory, and emotional changes associated with the menstrual cycle: a review. Arch Gynecol Obstet 2008;278:299–307.

Halbreich U. Algorithm for treatment of premenstrual syndromes (PMS): experts' recommendations and limitations. Gynecol Endocrinol 2005;20:48–56.

Herzog AG. Menstrual disorders in women with epilepsy. Neurology 2006;66(6 Suppl. 3):S23–8.

Jarvis CI, Lynch AM, Morin AK. Management strategies for premenstrual syndrome/premenstrual dysphoric disorder. Ann Pharmacother 2008;42:967–78.

Mannix LK, Files JA. The use of triptans in the management of menstrual migraine. CNS Drugs 2005;19:951–72.

Marjoribanks J, Proctor ML, Farquhar C. Nonsteroidal anti-inflammatory drugs for primary dysmenorrhoea. Cochrane Database Syst Rev 2003, Issue 4. Art. No.: CD001751.

Mattson RH, Cramer JA, Caldwell BV, Siconolfi BC. Treatment of seizures with medroxyprogesterone acetate: preliminary report. Neurology 1984;34:1255–8.

Mortola, JF, Girton, L, Beck, L, Yen, SSC. Diagnosis of premenstrual syndrome by a single, prospective and reliable instrument: the Calendar of Premenstrual Experiences. Obstet Gynecol 1990;76:302.

Proctor ML, Roberts H, Farquhar CM. Combined oral contraceptive pill (OCP) as treatment for primary dysmenorrhoea. Cochrane Database Syst Rev 2009, Issue 2. Art No.: CD002120.

Rapkin AJ, Winer SA. Premenstrual syndrome and premenstrual dysphoric disorder: quality of life and burden of illness. Expert Rev Pharmacoecon Outcomes Res 2009;9:157–70.

Reddy DS. Pharmacology of catamenial epilepsy. Methods Find Exp Clin Pharmacol 2004;26:547–61.

Redmond AM, James AW, Nolan SH, Self TH. Premenstrual asthma: emphasis on drug therapy options. J Asthma 2004;41:687–93.

Shah NR, Jones JB, Aperi J, Shemtov R, Karne A, Borenstein J. Selective serotonin reuptake inhibitors for premenstrual syndrome and premenstrual dysphoric disorder: a meta-analysis. Obstet Gynecol 2008;111:1175–82.

Silberstein SD, Merriam GR. Physiology of the menstrual cycle. Cephalalgia 2000;20:148–54.

Wyatt KM, Dimmock PW, O'Brien PM. Selective serotonin reuptake inhibitors for premenstrual syndrome. Cochrane Database Syst Rev 2009, Issue 2. Art. No.: CD001396.

Zarzycki W, Zieniewicz M. Reproductive disturbances in type 1 diabetic women. Neuro Endocrinol Lett 2005;26:733–8.

Irregular Bleeding During the Menopause Transition

Isiah D. Harris and William D. Schlaff

University of Colorado Health Sciences Center, Aurora, Colorado, USA

Dysfunctional uterine bleeding accounts for more than one third of gynecologic office visits. There is no period in a woman's life when unpredictable uterine bleeding occurs with greater frequency than during the menopausal transition. Most menstrual changes in the years before menopause are secondary to age-related anovulation, and the goal for clinicians is to distinguish normal physiology from the numerous potentially pathologic etiologies for altered menstrual patterns. While empiric treatments for anovulation are often successful, complete evaluation is warranted when the menstrual pattern is not consistent with typical menopause transition patterns of bleeding or when empiric therapies fail.

Definitions and epidemiology

The menopause transition begins at the point in a women's life when she experiences variations in the intermenstrual interval that are greater than 7 days from her normal cycle length, and ends 12 months after the last menstrual period. This definition is important to recognize because it has two important implications that affect clinical practice. The first is that the only objective measure to assess menopausal status is the menstrual pattern itself, and the utility of timed measurements of follicle-stimulating hormone (FSH), while interesting and occasionally insightful, is nondiagnostic. The second point is that irregularities in uterine bleeding patterns are a

normal part of aging for all women and are generally not pathologic. The fluctuation in intermenstrual cycle length is a result of a cessation of normal ovulation that occurs normally with aging (Figure 10.1).

The result of depleted ovarian reserve is an increased frequency of anovulatory cycles and oligomenorrhea, defined as menstrual cycles that last greater than 35 days or menses that occur fewer than eight times per year. Thus, a woman's menses can become more unpredictable, heavier, or prolonged. However, in addition to the normal fluctuations in the hypothalamic–pituitary–ovarian axis, women in the menopause transitional period have an increased incidence of polyps and fibroids. Therefore, if an abnormal bleeding persists following appropriate hormonal treatment of the oligomenorrhea, the clinician should consider the possibility of an anatomic lesion. Additionally, it must also be recognized that the increased frequency of oligo-ovulation means that women in the menopause transition have increased unopposed estrogen exposure, which increases the risk of endometrial hyperplasia and malignancy.

The average age of onset of the menopause transition is 46, and the average duration is 5 years. Ninety-five per cent of women will experience the onset of the transition between age 39 and 51, and will have a duration between 2–8 years in the transitional interval before the onset of menopause. The menopause transition occurs

Disorders of Menstruation, 1st edition. Edited by Paul B. Marshburn and Bradley S. Hurst.
© 2011 Blackwell Publishing Ltd.

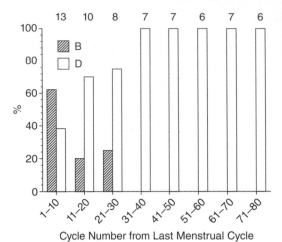

Figure 10.1 Percentage of long cycles (B) and normal cycles (D) in women approaching menopause. Reproduced from Landgren BM JCEM 2004.

earlier in Hispanic women and women who smoke, and occurs later in Japanese women and those who frequently consume alcohol. There is no correlation between onset of menopause and age of menarche, nor is menopause in any way associated with a history of oral contraceptive pill (OCP) usage. There is, however, a strong familial relationship such that women will typically undergo menstrual changes at a similar age to their mother or sisters.

Hormonal and menstrual changes

The normal menstrual cycle ranges between 24 and 35 days, but as women approach the menopause transition, generally in their late 30s and early 40s, they experience a shortening of their cycles that precedes the cycle lengthening that defines the transitional years. This menstrual change is directly related to an increase in the FSH level that occurs as a result of the accelerated loss of ovarian follicles that takes place in the menopause transition.

> ### ⚙ SCIENCE REVISITED
>
> Women are born with 1–2 million oocytes, and have approximately 300,000–500,000 remaining at puberty. Over the reproductive years, 400–500 of these oocytes will be

selected for natural ovulation, and the number of remaining follicles slowly declines until late in the fourth decade of life, when it is about 25,000. Beyond this threshold, the rate of follicular loss is accelerated, and the remaining follicles are of poor quality such that the granulosa cells of these follicles are less effective at producing inhibin. Inhibin is the primary source of negative feedback signaling from the ovary to the anterior pituitary and, in conjunction with estradiol, functions to limit the secretion of follicle-stimulating hormone (FSH). As inhibin levels fall in transitional women, the FSH levels rise concordantly and there is earlier follicular recruitment and dominant follicle selection, earlier maturation of the dominant follicle, and a shorter follicular phase.

The length of the luteal phase may remain constant, and thus the menstrual cycle is shortened, with the average women experiencing a nadir in her menstrual cycle length at age 42. Alternately, poor follicular development may be associated with blunted hormonal secretion from the follicle, poor corpus luteum formation, and a shortened luteal phase. Thereafter, there is a gradual increase in cycle length and variability that is the hallmark of the menopausal transition.

There is a common misconception regarding estradiol levels during the menopause transition. As previously mentioned, inhibin serves as the primary negative feedback stimulus for FSH production, so despite rising FSH levels during this time, estradiol levels are typically unchanged and may in fact be slightly elevated in the early transitional period. It is not until near-complete depletion of resting oocytes has occurred that estrogen levels decline, and they do so rapidly in the final year prior to menopause. Therefore, early follicular phase assessment of estradiol levels is usually not an informative marker of oocyte depletion and should not be used for this purpose. Similarly, while FSH levels rise steadily throughout the menopause transition, there is no threshold value that can diagnose or prognosticate the timing of menopause. Generally, FSH levels will rise slowly to about 20 IU/L and then

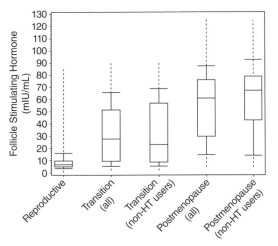

Figure 10.2 Follicle-stimulating hormone levels in menopause transition. HT, hormone therapy. Reproduced from Henrick JB et al Menopause 2006.

thereafter begin a more rapid increase over 1–3 years to typical menopausal levels, which are greater than 50 IU/L (Figure 10.2). One must keep in mind that these values are gross generalizations and should not be considered diagnostic because low values are often misleading.

Endocrinopathies that cause abnormal uterine bleeding

When women present with a menopause transitional bleeding pattern, it is important to evaluate for other potential endocrine abnormalities that frequently occur in this age group. Hypothyroidism is diagnosed with increasing frequency with age, and the prevalence in women is high enough that screening is recommended every 5 years after age 35. Indeed, some suggest increasing the frequency of screening to every 2 years after age 60. Women are five to eight times more likely to have thyroid dysfunction than men, and 15% of older women will have positive antithyroid antibodies. In considering the primary care of the woman during the menopause transitional years, evaluation of thyroid function is a critical component of healthcare maintenance and has specific implications as regards menstrual function.

Menstrual irregularities are more commonly associated with hypothyroidism than hyperthy-roidism. Thyrotropin-releasing hormone produced in the hypothalamus acts on the anterior pituitary to stimulate the release of thyroid-stimulating hormone (TSH). TSH then acts directly on the thyroid to produce thyroxine (T4) and triiodothyronine (T3), which enter the circulation and are 70% bound to thyroid-binding globulin and 30% bound to albumin or prealbumin. T4 has greater affinity for binding, and therefore it is T3 that more readily enters the peripheral cells and has direct effects. However, in the pituitary and the brain, T4 is readily taken up and can be converted intracellularly to T3, so serum concentrations of T4 and TSH are the best markers of overall thyroid function.

SCIENCE REVISITED

Thyroid-binding globulin (TBG) is synthesized by the liver, and its rate of synthesis is increased by circulating estrogen, whether endogenous or exogenous. Increased TBG will result in increased total thyroxine (T4) levels, although free T4 levels are unchanged. Thyrotropin-releasing hormone (TRH) also has receptors on prolactin-secreting cells in the pituitary and stimulates prolactin secretion. In patients with primary hypothyroidism, the thyroid gland is unable to produce sufficient quantities of T4 in response to normal thyroid-stimulating hormone (TSH) levels, usually related to autoimmune disease such as Hashimoto thyroiditis. In response to falling T4 levels, the hypothalamus increases TRH production, which secondarily increases TSH production in the pituitary to drive higher levels of T4 production. In this state, the elevated TRH activity secondarily increases prolactin production, which interferes with the gonadatropin-releasing hormone pulse generator. The pulsatile secretion of follicle-stimulating hormone and luteinizing hormone required for normal menstruation is thereby suppressed, resulting in diminished circulating levels of gonadotropins. As a result, hypothyroid women will typically have anovulatory cycles and present with amenorrhea or oligomenorrhea.

Simple thyroid replacement with levothyroxine will reverse the gonadotropin-releasing hormone (GnRH) pulse generator defect and typically result in resolution of normal menstruation within 1–2 months of achieving a euthyroid state. It is useful to note that while subclinical hypothyroidism has a prevalence of up to 10% in middle-aged and elderly women, it is not typically responsible for dysfunctional uterine bleeding. Subclinical hypothyroidism should be treated as it is associated with dyslipidemia and may increase the risk for development of coronary artery disease. It is also implicated for women experiencing recurrent miscarriage, a common problem in older women trying to conceive. However, treatment of subclinical hypothyroidism is unlikely to improve dysfunctional uterine bleeding, and an alternative etiology should be pursued.

The mechanism by which hyperthyroid women develop menstrual dysfunction is unclear. The two most prevalent causes of hyperthyroidism are Graves disease and Plummer disease, both of which are uncommonly associated with amenorrhea and oligomenorrhea.

Prolactin secretion occurs not only in the lactotrophs of the anterior pituitary gland, but also in decidualized endometrial tissue and in the myometrium. These different sites have separate regulatory mechanisms and, as mentioned in the above discussion of hypothyroidism, hyperprolactinemia results in impairment of the GnRH pulse generator and thereby causes anovulation.

Mechanical causes of bleeding

As mentioned previously, the development of an anovulatory bleeding pattern during menopause transition is an anticipated event, but women are also at risk for anatomic abnormalities during this time, which can result in abnormal uterine bleeding. A careful menstrual history can often increase the suspicion for or effectively rule out anatomic etiologies of abnormal uterine bleeding. In women whose primary complaint is menorrhagia despite a regular menstrual interval, or persistent intermenstrual bleeding, or who fail traditional empiric therapies for anovulatory bleeding patterns, further evaluation for ana-

tomic causes should be pursued as outlined in Chapters 6 and 7.

Polyps

As described in Chapter 6, endometrial polyps can cause vascular fragility, chronic intrauterine inflammation, and endometrial surface erosions that result in abnormal uterine bleeding. The typical bleeding profile of women with endometrial polyps is recurrent intermenstrual bleeding. It is rare that polyps are discovered before age 20, and the incidence increases steadily with age, with the peak incidence occurring in the menopause transition. The reason for the increased susceptibility has not been determined but likely relates to the hyperestrogenic state that defines this stage of life.

Endometrial polyps are discovered in 10–24% of endometrial biopsy samples but are rarely associated with malignancy. In fact, less than 1% of polyps harbor an underlying neoplasm. This is particularly pertinent for women during the menopause transition because they will often have incidental findings of small polyps on radiographic imaging or biopsy samples for a history of abnormal bleeding. Incidentally discovered polyps do not require removal during the transitional years unless they exceed 2 cm in size or unless the woman has other risk factors for malignancy such as obesity, tamoxifen use, estrogen monotherapy, chronic anovulation, or a personal or family history of ovarian, breast, colon, or endometrial cancer. Certainly, polyps that are symptomatic for metrorrhagia or menorrhagia should be removed, but asymptomatic polyps, including those discovered in patients with new-onset anovulatory bleeding patterns, are likely to spontaneously regress over a 2–3-year period.

Fibroids

The hyperestrogenic environment associate with menopause transition is often considered a cause for increased growth of pre-existing leiomyomas; however, the specific mechanisms for fibroid growth are unclear. In fact, fibroids typically grow at a slower rate after age 35 in Caucasian but not African-American women. As previously discussed in Chapter 6, submucous fibroids are a common and benign cause of menorrhagia for many women, but particularly affect younger, African-American women. However, clinically relevant fibroids, defined as those greater than 4 cm in size or those in a submucous location on transvaginal ultrasonography, are present in over 50% of African-American women and over 35% of Caucasian women during the menopause transition.

Adenomyosis

Adenomyosis is a condition involving the presence of endometrial glands and stroma within the myometrium, and results in a bulky or enlarged uterus. The two most common symptoms of this condition are dysmenorrhea and menorrhagia. Because the diagnosis of adenomyosis can only be made definitively by pathologic investigation at the time of hysterectomy, the clinical incidence is difficult to determine, although it is generally considered to affect approximately 20% of women. Despite being a pathologic diagnosis, adenomyosis can be suggested on imaging studies. Transvaginal ultrasound has a sensitivity and specificity approaching 85% in some studies. Magnetic resonance imaging (MRI) is superior to ultrasound, although significantly more expensive. For patients in whom adenomyosis is suspected and in whom empiric medical treatments have failed, surgical intervention is more likely to be beneficial than MRI for abnormal uterine bleeding. The available surgical techniques are described later in this chapter.

The relationship of adenomyosis to age or menopause transitional status is unclear. The incidence is presumed to increase with age as risk factors include parity and prior uterine surgery, both of which affect a greater absolute number of women as age progresses beyond the third decade of life.

Chronic endometritis

Inflammatory mediators are a normal part of the process of menstruation. However, when the endometrium becomes chronically inflamed and proteolytic enzymes predominate, the result is a disrupted subepithelial capillary plexus and surface epithelium. This insult to the normal architecture of the endometrium renders it fragile and susceptible to erosion. Furthermore, the inflamed state impairs the normal repair processes of the menstrual cycle and thereby can present with persistent, heavy, or irregularly timed bleeding. Inflammation may result from the presence of a foreign body such as an intrauterine contraceptive device (IUD), but also plays a significant role in the bleeding patterns of women with either fibroids or polyps. Obviously, infection is an important cause of inflammation, and women during the menopause transition are as susceptible to ascending sexually transmitted infections as younger women, although screening for sexually transmitted infections is often overlooked in this age group. In addition to performing endocervical cultures for such infections, women who have plasma cells noted on an endometrial biopsy sample should have that sample cultured. It should be noted, however, that the majority of chronic endometritis caused by infection is actually a result of common vaginal flora bacteria or *Mycoplasma* and is not associated with sexually transmitted infection.

Tuberculous endometritis should be considered in women who come from countries where tuberculosis is endemic and in those who may not have had access to effective chemoprophylaxis despite living in developed countries. These women will often have complaints of vague pelvic or abdominal pain, and many will have associated renal involvement. Diagnosis should start with purified protein derivative tuberculin skin testing and a chest radiograph to assess for healed granulomas, although imaging will be normal most patients. The diagnosis confirmed by histologic evaluation of a surgical specimen showing granulomas, or through acid-fast bacillus testing or culture of menstrual blood or an endometrial biopsy sample. The most sensitive test is actually culture of menstrual blood collected in a vaginal or cervical cup, but all of these tests are useful in making the diagnosis in cases with a high suspicion.

Treatments

Menopausal transition-associated anovulatory bleeding is a diagnosis of exclusion. A careful menstrual history will often be sufficient to allow initiation of empiric treatment, but the complete differential diagnosis must be carefully considered and other etiologies pursued if initial empiric therapies fail.

Nonsteroidal anti-inflammatory drugs

Nonsteroidal anti-inflammatory drugs (NSAIDs) are a commonly prescribed and safe family of medications that are often useful for the control of menorrhagia. By modulating the effects of prostaglandins on the endometrial vascular homeostatic mechanisms, NSAIDs can reduce menstrual blood flow by 20–40%. Although the most studied medications for this indication are mefenamic acid and the closely related anti-fibrinolytic agent tranexamic acid, these are prohibitively expensive for most patients, and naproxen is likely just as effective and a better first-line choice. When prescribed for menorrhagia, treatment should begin with the onset of bleeding and continue for 3–5 days depending on cycle length. Although effective for menorrhagia, the heavy bleeding associated with the menopause transition is usually best treated with hormonal therapy.

Oral contraceptive pill

Despite being combination pills, all OCPs are progestin dominant and are therefore highly effective for the management of anovulatory bleeding during the menopause transition. These can be taken in the traditional cyclic fashion or, preferentially for many women, in a continuous fashion where withdrawal bleeding is induced every 3–4 months. Additionally, there is evidence to suggest that shortening the placebo-pill interval from 7 days to 4 days will further reduce the amount of menstrual flow and decrease the risks for intermenstrual spotting that commonly occurs with extended-cycle OCP use.

Despite being highly effective, OCPs are significantly underutilized in the menopause transition population. This is likely due to fears of both patients and providers relating to potential adverse consequences of hormone therapy in women over age 35, most notably the risk of thromboembolic disease. It is certainly true that the risk of thromboembolic disease increases with age in both men and women, and it is also true that exogenous estrogen increases the risk of thromboembolism and cardiovascular mortality. However, it is important to balance the absolute impact of OCPs, particularly in light of other risk factors and the risks associated with no treatment.

For nonsmokers over age 35, the cardiovascular disease mortality risk is increased from 3.2 to 6.2 deaths per 100,000 woman–years. Although this can be stated as doubling the risk of cardiovascular disease-related death, the absolute risk is still extremely small. For light smokers, defined as those who smoke fewer than 10 cigarettes per day, the literature does not support any significant increase in risk. In fact, even though a synergistic effect exists between OCP use and heavy smoking, the use of OCPs in heavy-smoking women increases the risk of cardiovascular related death from 10 to 29 per 100,000 woman–years, again a large relative increase, but a very small absolute risk. The risks of fatal thromboembolic disease or cerebrovascular accident are comparable to those for cardiovascular-related death. When compared to the risks associated with pregnancy, which are only slightly lower, the importance of birth control to avoid unintended pregnancy cannot be overstated.

> ### ✋ CAUTION
>
> Given these risks, it is prudent for women to be carefully counseled about the potential risks of oral contraceptive pills during the transitional years and the impact of reversible risk factors such as obesity and smoking. As providers, it is also important to recognize that not all oral contraceptives are equal with respect to their risk profiles. While providers appropriately seek to use the lowest dosage forms of estrogen available, the impact of the progestagen component is also important and often overlooked. First-generation progestagens such as norethindrone or ethynodiol have the lowest risk for thromboembolic disease, and the second-generation progestagens (norgestrel, levonorgestrel) are similarly safe. However, there is ample evidence that the third-generation progestagens containing desogesterel place women at increased risk for thromboembolic events. This is particularly

relevant because some of the commonly used, low-dose estrogen pills containing between 20 and 30 µg ethinylestradiol are combined with a third-generation progestagen and should probably be avoided in this cohort.

Progesterone-only pills and the levonorgestrel-secreting intrauterine device

Because combined OCP therapy does pose increased risks, it important that we recognize that a safe and effective alternative exists. The progestin-only pills (POPs) that are commercially available and approved for contraception are norethindrone formulations. This first-generation progestagen avoids the thromboembolic and cardiac safety risks of combined pills and is safe as monotherapy even in patients at high thromboembolic risk. The risk of POP use is reduced efficacy as birth control (an approximately 8% failure rate with typical use versus 3% with combined OCPs) and an increased risk of unscheduled or breakthrough bleeding.

Understandably, breakthrough bleeding is a significant adverse reaction when the goal of therapy is to treat abnormal uterine bleeding. To minimize this risk, progestagens such as medroxyprogesterone acetate or norethindrone acetate can be used in a cyclic fashion. The goal of cyclic therapy is to mimic the corpus luteum and provide an organized withdrawal bleed every 1–2 months to prevent the endometrial overgrowth and disorganized breakdown typical of anovulatory women.

> ### ☆ TIPS & TRICKS
>
> We recommend that patients be treated with a total of 50–70 mg medroxyprogesterone acetate every 1–2 months, divided over a course of 7–10 consecutive days. Timing of therapy does not need to be correlated with natural cycles and can be fixed to a calendar (the most convenient being the first 7–10 days of every month or every other month).

> ### ☒ CAUTION
>
> It is crucial to note that neither medroxyprogesterone acetate nor norethindrone acetate functions as birth control when used in the cyclic fashion described, and therefore another form of birth control should be used concomitantly depending on the patient's circumstances. It should also be made clear to patients that using oral contraceptive pills in this fashion may result in intermenstrual bleeding associated with a natural ovulation and progesterone withdrawal.

For those women who are amenable to the levonorgestrel IUD, there are several advantages compared to either OCPs or POPs. First, the IUD provides superior birth control, with a failure rate of less than 1%. Second, it provides for long-term treatment. Since the average duration of the menopause transition is 5 years, most women can be effectively managed through this transition with a single treatment with the levonorgestrel-secreting IUD which is approved by the Food and Drug Administration for 5 years of use, but has been proven to have efficacy up to 7 years. Third, it avoids estrogen exposure for high-risk patients or those particularly nervous about the thromboembolic or cardiac risks of systemic estrogen therapy. Fourth, it provides optimal endometrial protection for patients at high risk for endometrial hyperplasia and malignancy, and it is in fact a recommended treatment for hyperplasia or low-grade malignancy in patients who are poor surgical candidates. Finally, it reduces menstrual blood flow to the greatest degree, by about 80% in most patients, with 20% of patients having complete amenorrhea after 1 year. Patients are generally more satisfied with the IUD than POPs, despite the fact that both have the risk of unscheduled or breakthrough bleeding, although this is generally very light and of short duration.

Gonadotropin-releasing hormone agonists

GnRH agonists are a safe and effective treatment for women with irregular or heavy bleeding, although they are rarely employed for this indication given the availability of other effective and less expensive options that have much fewer side effects. GnRH agonists are initially stimulatory on the anterior pituitary production of FSH and luteinizing hormone (LH), but after a period of 7–10 days of constant exposure the GnRH receptors are down-regulated and become uncoupled from their second messenger systems. Thereafter, FSH and LH levels are significantly reduced, resulting in a hypoestrogenic state and eliminating endometrial proliferation. Side effects include those commonly associated with menopause, such as hot flashes, vaginal dryness, mild cognitive impairment, emotional lability, and sleep disturbances. Not all women experience these symptoms to the same degree, and some are completely undisturbed by the medication, but the vast majority will have some level of side effects. These effects can be managed with concomitant use of hormonal add-back including low-dose estrogen, progestin, or a combination of both.

The most common use for GnRH agonists in women during the transitional years is in the management of uterine fibroids. GnRH agonists are generally effective in reducing the size of fibroids, although the level of reduction in the size of myomas is quite variable. Nevertheless, this approach is often effective in reducing or eliminating abnormal bleeding. Women who have intracavitary myomas will often have a lower reduction in vaginal bleeding. More significant is the utility of GnRH agonist pretreatment in preoperative planning for definitive surgery such as hysterectomy. Studies have shown that 3 months of GnRH agonist treatment coupled with iron therapy will significantly improve hemoglobin levels in anemic women. Additionally, preoperative GnRH agonist treatment is associated with reduced operative blood loss and may permit a less invasive surgical approach. Many surgeons claim that the use of a GnRH agonist prior to myomectomy may impair the identification of surgical planes along the pseudocapsule, making the procedure more difficult. This, however, has not been established in the available literature and remains anecdotal.

High dose estrogen

Although counterintuitive, high-dose estrogen therapy can be a highly effective therapy for women who present with menorrhagia and significant anemia during the menopause transition. For the majority of women with hyperplastic endometrium related to chronic anovulation, progestin therapy is the best choice. However, women with severely denuded or attenuated endometrial linings will also occasionally present with severe menorrhagia, and these women are best treated with high-dose estrogen therapy. Transvaginal ultrasound is very useful at distinguishing women with a thick endometrial stripe (>10 mm), in whom disordered shedding of the endometrial lining will respond best to progestin therapy or OCPs, from those women with a markedly thin endometrial lining (<5 mm), for whom estrogen therapy should be more effective. Treatment can be given orally with either 1.25 mg of conjugated estrogens or 2.0 mg of micronized estradiol, every 4–6 hours for up to 24 hours; alternatively, in emergent cases or patients who require inpatient observation, intravenous therapy can be given, with 25 mg of conjugated estrogen therapy every 6–12 hours for up to 24 hours. After initial treatment, therapy should be tapered to a once-daily oral dose for an additional 7–10 days, and patients can be maintained thereafter on OCPs.

Surgery

For women in whom anatomic pathology is identified and medical management fails or is undesirable because of medical concerns or the patient's personal reasons, surgery is a reasonable alternative. There are a number of different procedures that are reviewed in an earlier chapter, but these briefly include uterine artery embolization, dilatation and curettage, endometrial ablation, and hysterectomy.

Women should be counseled toward the least invasive option that has a reasonable chance of achieving treatment goals. For many women, this will mean undergoing an endometrial ablation procedure through one of several available methods. This procedure is associated with up to an 80% reduction in bleeding, and over 80% of women will continue to be satisfied after 5 years, again paralleling the average duration of the menopause transition and after which bleeding will natural subside.

There has been some concern raised about the theoretical possibility of creating islands of functional endometrial tissue beneath the eschar of the ablated endometrial surface. These functional islands could potentially then develop into endometrial cancers that might not be recognized until a late stage since these women will not have abnormal uterine bleeding. For this reason, it is recommended that all women have an endometrial biopsy or dilatation or curettage performed prior to or at the same time as an ablative procedure. While some recommend that women at high risk for endometrial hyperplasia or malignancy do not undergo endometrial ablation, there has been no evidence to date to suggest that the theoretical risk of hiding a future malignancy has any clinical merit. As always, appropriate and thorough counseling is of pre-eminent importance, but having risk factors for endometrial cancer is not an absolute contraindication to endometrial ablation.

Pregnancy and fertility

The decreased use of OCPs secondary to thromboembolic concerns is a major contributor to unintended pregnancies during the menopause transition. Additionally, many women believe that they cannot get pregnant after age 40 or 45 and therefore do not make contraception a priority.

A classic study of natural fertility in the Hutterite community revealed that although fertility rates decline, often rapidly, after age 35, the potential for fertility exists until the age of menopause. The fertility rate of a 40-year-old woman is about 5% per month, and the oldest women to conceive spontaneously was over 57 years old. Over 50% of pregnancies in women over age 40 are unintended, and 65% of these result in elective termination.

It is important to remember that the most common etiology for a sudden departure from a pattern of regularly timed menstrual cycles is in fact pregnancy, and women need to have a birth control method in place to protect against the burden of unplanned pregnancy until menopausal.

While birth control is a major concern for many women during the transitional years, others in this age group will, however, present desiring fertility treatments and evaluation. Infertility is defined as the inability to conceive despite greater than 12 months of unprotected intercourse. Approximately 50% of couples with normal fertility will conceive within 3 months of trying, 75% will conceive within 6 months, and 85% of couples will have conceived within a year. This means that, for couples who have not conceived over a 6-month period of time, over half will fail to conceive over the following 6 months and will meet the definition of infertility. Furthermore, the fertility potential of women generally begins a rapid decline after age 35, and there is increasing likelihood of poor oocyte quality and quantity, otherwise referred to as diminished ovarian reserve.

Given that conception rate declines with age, a fertility evaluation and treatment for women over age 35 should be initiated after a period of 6 months without successful conception. Women over age 40 are encouraged to seek fertility assessment as soon as they are considering conception.

Infertility testing typically begins with serum screening on the third day of the menstrual cycle, although screening on days 2 or 4 is similarly accurate. The best studied test for ovarian reserve is FSH, which should be in the range of 5–10 mIU/mL. Values of 10–15 mIU/mL suggest diminished ovarian reserve, and values above this threshold are consistent with severely diminished ovarian reserve and are suggestive of, although not diagnostic for, the menopause transition. Occasionally, patients will present with values less than 5 mIU/mL. In these cases, consideration should be given to the possibility of hypogonadotropic hypogonadism, which is a primary deficiency in the pituitary production of FSH. Although this condition is clinically significant and not uncommon, it presents in early reproductive life and is not a likely diagnosis during the menopause transition.

★ TIPS & TRICKS

We check an estradiol value and generally counsel patients that normal values are below 60 pg/mL. Values between 60 and 80 pg/mL are borderline, and values above 80 pg/mL are abnormal. In addition, we recommend measurement of antimüllerian hormone to further estimate the quality of remaining oocytes and the quantitative ovarian reserve. Like inhibin, this hormone is produced by the granulosa cells of the antral follicles. Therefore, the more follicles there are and the more efficient the granulosa cells, the higher this value will be. This hormone is relatively new in the assessment of ovarian reserve, and the specific thresholds of normal and abnormal are still debated. We generally counsel patients that values greater than 2 ng/mL are normal, values between 1 and 2 ng/mL are borderline, and values less than 1 ng/mL are reflective of diminished ovarian reserve. Some authors and clinicians suggest that antimüllerian hormone should and will supplant follicle-stimulating hormone as the "gold standard" ovarian reserve test, but additional evidence and experience are required at present.

★ TIPS & TRICKS

We generally perform an ultrasound on day 2, 3, or 4 of the cycle to assess for the presence of uterine pathology and to evaluate the number of small antral follicles (2–8 mm in size) remaining in the ovary. Diminished ovarian function is associated with depletion of antral follicles.

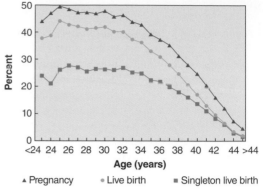

▲ Pregnancy   ● Live birth   ■ Singleton live birth

*For consistency all percentages are based on cycles started.

Figure 10.3 Age-related decline in pregnancy after in-vitro fertilization. Reproduced from CDEC.

Random blood draw for TSH to assess for thyroid function and prolactin to rule out hyperprolactinemia is also recommended. Depending on the patient's history, a hysterosalpingogram may be indicated to assess the uterine cavity as well as to determine the patency of the fallopian tubes. In some cases in which patients have a history suggestive of endometriosis or peritoneal adhesive disease, a laparoscopy is recommended to evaluate the peritoneal cavity and eliminate disease affecting the ovaries or fallopian tubes. The evaluation of women seeking fertility during the menopause transition will depend on their overall prognosis for success based on an evaluation of ovarian function. Further evaluation may not be indicated if ovarian reserve testing shows an extremely poor prognosis; referral for oocyte or embryo donation may be appropriate for healthy women who wish to consider these options (Figure 10.3).

Endometrial hyperplasia and malignancy

Endometrial cancer is the most common gynecologic malignancy in the United States, while cervical cancer is the most common worldwide. Although endometrial cancer occurs predominately in postmenopausal women, 25% of cases are diagnosed in women during the menopause transition, and up to 10% of these occur in women under the age of 40.

SCIENCE REVISITED

Women have a 2.5% lifetime risk of developing endometrial cancer, and although it develops in Caucasians more frequently than African-Americans, African-American women have a twofold risk of mortality secondary to issues related to access to care and differences in cancer subtypes between the two ethnic groups. The two subtypes of endometrial cancer are distinguished by histopathology and relation to estrogen. Type I is the common subtype, occurring in about 80% of endometrial cancers, comprises typically low-grade endometroid tumors, and is related to endometrial hyperplasia and unopposed estrogen exposure. Type II endometrial cancer occur in only 20% of cases but disproportionately affects African-American women. These carcinomas are typically unrelated to estrogen exposure and represent higher-grade tumors such as papillary serous or clear cell histology.

Risk factors

There are several known risk factors for development of endometrial cancer, all of which relate specifically to type I endometrial cancer. The most pertinent of these for women during the menopause transition is the unopposed estrogen exposure related to a history of chronic anovulation. Despite not having normal follicular development and ovarian estrogen production, these women have normal androgen levels, and peripheral conversion of androgen to estrogen allows for normal to elevated systemic estrogen levels. With persistent exposure to estrogen without corpus luteal development and associated progesterone secretion, the endometrial lining is chronically stimulated to proliferate. Over time, this can lead to hyperplasia and possibly malignancy.

Adipose cells are the primary site of aromatization of androgens to estradiol, and through this mechanism obese women have higher endogenous estrogen levels and higher risk for hyperplasia and malignancy. This is further exacerbated by lower levels of sex hormone-binding globulin and higher rates of insulin resistance. Consistent with the mechanisms described above, other well-established risk factors include obesity, diabetes, tamoxifen use, nulliparity, and alcohol use.

Protective factors

Several studies have assessed a plethora of possible protective factors against the development of endometrial cancer. Among the proposed protective factors, many are counterintuitive. For example, smoking has been associated with a 30% reduction in risk of developing endometrial cancer, but this protective effect clearly is outweighed by the myriad other health risks of smoking. Furthermore, the protective effect of smoking does not apply to women during the menopause transition.

Coffee use has also been associated with a reduced endometrial cancer risk, with heavier coffee drinkers having a greater protective effect. Some limited evidence suggests that increased physical activity is also protective, although this relationship is not conclusive. Finally, OCP use and combined hormone replacement therapy are protective, as they provide progesterone protection to the endometrium.

These risk factors are important to appreciate in considering investigation for endometrial cancer in the transitional period. As discussed in the opening of this chapter, an anovulatory bleeding pattern is to be expected during the menopause transition. However, the American College of Obstetrics and Gynecology recommends that any woman over age 35 with greater than 6 months of oligomenorrhea warrants evaluation for endometrial cancer. Although strict adherence to this recommendation inevitably leads to unnecessary evaluations in very low-risk women, endometrial biopsy is an uncomfortable but low-risk intervention. Other indications for biopsy include women found to have atypical endometrial cells on a Papanicolau smear, although physiologic shedding of normal-appearing endometrial cells is not a concerning finding. Finally, women under age 35 with multiple risk factors and irregular bleeding should also be screened.

Screening and diagnosis

Screening for endometrial cancer is only recommended for women with a personal or family history of hereditary nonpolyposis colorectal cancer. These women have an approximately 50% lifetime risk of developing endometrial cancer, and therefore screening has been recommended to start at age 35 with annual endometrial biopsy. Otherwise, there are no populations for which screening of asymptomatic women with either endometrial sampling or ultrasound is recommended, including women using tamoxifen.

> ### ⚠ CAUTION
>
> For women who warrant assessment for possible malignancy, the options for assessment include endometrial sampling versus imaging. Although ultrasound or sonohysterography is useful for the evaluation of the benign etiologies of abnormal uterine bleeding, they are not useful for ruling out malignancy in women before menopause. It is not unusual for a woman to have an endometrial stripe 10 mm or more during the transitional years, which is distinct from the postmenopausal woman. Similarly, although hysteroscopy is a useful tool in assessing the endometrial cavity and can increase or decrease the suspicion for endometrial pathology, it cannot definitively diagnose or rule out malignancy.

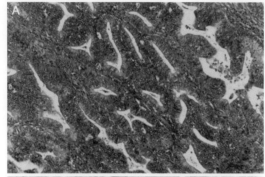
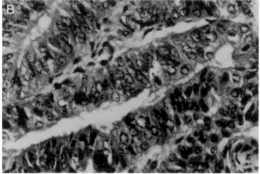

Figure 10.4 Endometrial hypoplasia. Reproduced from Montgomery BE Obstet Gynecol Surv 2004.

Therefore, in this population, malignancy can only be reasonably assessed with endometrial sampling. In this respect, there has not been shown to be any significant difference between endometrial biopsy with a 3 mm Pipelle and dilatation and curettage. Thus, it is recommended that patients have an in-office biopsy for increased ease of scheduling and lower cost. Additionally, with a normal office biopsy result, patients can be reassured.

However, for patients with evidence of hyperplasia or who have persistently abnormal bleeding despite treatment, further evaluation is warranted. Hyperplasia is identified as either simple or complex. These biopsy samples are further assessed for the presence or absence of atypical features. There is increased risk of developing malignancy when a biopsy sample shows evidence of complexity, and even greater risk when atypical features are present (Figure 10.4). Furthermore, there is evidence to suggest that endometrial biopsy and dilatation and curettage will underestimate the severity of endometrial pathology. Therefore, when hyperplasia is present on an endometrial biopsy sample, women should be offered dilatation and curettage with diagnostic hysteroscopy to definitively rule out an occult malignancy. Any women in whom malignancy is confirmed should have referral to a gynecologic oncologist for further management.

Alternatively, for women with hyperplasia who are not interested in future childbearing during the menopause transition, definitive surgery with hysterectomy should be considered. For those who are interested in future childbearing, are poor surgical candidates, or do not have atypical features, medical management can be considered. High-dose progestin therapy is the treatment of choice, and either oral treatment or local therapy with an IUD is effective.

Selected bibliography

Day Baird D, Dunson DB, Hill MC, Cousins D, Schectman JM. High cumulative incidence of uterine leiomyoma in black and white women: ultrasound evidence. Am J Obstet Gynecol 2003;188:100–7.

Kurman RJ, Kaminski PF, Norris HJ. The behavior of endometrial hyperplasia. A long term study of "untreated" hyperplasia in 170 patients. Cancer 1985;56:403–12.

Lethaby A, Vollenhoven B, Swoter MC. Preoperative GNRH analogue therapy for hysterectomy or myomectomy for uterine fibroids (Review). Cochrane Database Syst Rev 2001, Issue 2. Art. No.: CD000547.

Meredith SM, Sanchez-Ramos L, Kaunitz AM. Diagnostic accuracy of transvaginal sonography for the diagnosis of adenomyosis: systematic review and metaanalysis. Am J Obstet Gynecol 2009;201:107.e1–6.

Peddada SD, Laughlin SK, Miner K et al. Growth of uterine leiomyomata among premenopausal black and white women. Proc Natl Acad Sci U S A 2008;105:19887–92.

Schwingl PJ, Ory HW, Visness CM. Estimates of the risk of cardiovascular death attributable to low-dose oral contraceptives in the United States. Am J Obstet Gynecol 1999;180(1 Pt 1):241–9.

Suh-Burgmann E, Hung YY, Armstrong MA. Complex atypical hyperplasia: the risk of unrecognized adenocarcinoma and the value of preoperative dilation and curettage. Obstet Gynecol 2009;114:523–9.

Thonneau P, Goulard H, Goyaux N. Risk factors for intrauterine device failure: a review. Contraception 200;64:33–7.

Postmenopausal Bleeding

Karen D. Bradshaw[1] and David Tait[2]

[1]University of Texas Southwestern Medical Center at Dallas, Dallas, Texas, USA
[2]Carolinas Medical Center, Charlotte, North Carolina, USA

Introduction

Menopause refers to a woman's last menstrual period and is caused by the permanent cessation of ovulation. Since menses can be infrequent during the menopause transition, the time of menopause can only be determined after a woman has experienced 12 months without menstrual bleeding.

Menopause can occur at any age, with a median age of 51.5 years. Approximately 10% of women by age 45, 80% of women by age 52, 95% of women by age 55, and nearly 100% of women by age 58 have reached menopause. Because bleeding is the presenting sign in more than 90% of patients with endometrial cancer, any bleeding after 12 months of amenorrhea in a postmenopausal woman warrants immediate evaluation, no matter how scant or episodic the bleeding. The true incidence of postmenopausal bleeding decreases with age, but the probability of cancer being the cause increases from 9% for patients in their 50s to 60% in their 80s.

> ✋ CAUTION!
>
> Any bleeding that occurs in postmenopausal women is considered "cancer until proven otherwise," although the incidence of malignancy in such patients ranges from 4% to 24%, depending on risk factors.

Postmenopausal women taking hormone treatment should be evaluated in the same manner as patients not using hormone therapy as they have similar risks for endometrial cancer. Postmenopausal women with abnormal vaginal staining, odor, or heavy vaginal discharge should be evaluated for endometrial cancer.

The role of the clinician for women who present with bleeding is twofold: to exclude endometrial cancer and to identify any source of benign bleeding so it can be stopped or managed. Hormone therapy is associated with unscheduled bleeding or spotting in up to 40% of women using therapy, due to effects of the hormones, atrophic or disordered endometrium, and intracavitary lesions. The majority of postmenopausal bleeding in all women is due to atrophy of the endometrium or vagina (40–50%), endometrial cancer (10%), and polyps (3%). Evaluation of postmenopausal bleeding can be done quickly and efficiently.

History and physical examination

An accurate patient history is fundamental in diagnosing postmenopausal bleeding. Specific hormonal, medical, and age-related risk factors significantly increase a woman's chance of having reproductive tract cancer, and astute clinicians will question patients accordingly. A short list of differential diagnosis exists for postmenopausal bleeding, and with a thorough, targeted history,

Disorders of Menstruation, 1st edition. Edited by Paul B. Marshburn and Bradley S. Hurst.
© 2011 Blackwell Publishing Ltd.

physical examination, pelvic examination, and imaging with transvaginal ultrasonography (TVUS), as well as possible targeted endometrial biopsy, the etiology of the postmenopausal bleeding can be determined in the initial visit if sonography is available.

The history should focus on the most likely causes of abnormal bleeding and establish its initial onset, amount, and frequency. Identified risk factors for endometrial carcinoma include increasing age, obesity, diabetes, unopposed estrogen or tamoxifen use, and polycystic ovarian syndrome. These risk factors share common pathways of estrogenic stimulation of the endometrium through increasing extraglandular conversion of steroid precursors to estrogen by up-regulation of the aromatase enzyme in adipose tissue, or by direct estrogen stimulation of the endometrium. In contrast, postmenopausal women with breast cancer taking oral aromatase inhibitors such as letrozole or anastrazole that are antiestrogenic in the breast and endometrium are more likely to bleed from endometrial atrophy.

A family history of uterine, breast, ovarian, or colon cancer may increase the risk for endometrial cancer. Symptoms of bloating, early satiety, pelvic pain and/or pressure, and pelvic floor descent should be investigated as these may indicate the presence of uterine pathology or other disorders, including ovarian cancer.

> ### ☆ TIPS AND TRICKS
>
> The physician should ensure that bleeding is from the genital tract, and not be confused by urologic or gastrointestinal bleeding, which require appropriate referral. Symptoms of urinary frequency, dysuria, or recent urinary tract infection should be elicited. Bleeding with passage of feces, after bowel movements, or after wiping on sanitary products could be associated with external or internal hemorrhoids, anal fissures, polyps, or anal or gastrointestinal cancers. In most cases, identification of blood on the cervical aspect of a tampon confirms the presence of bleeding from the reproductive tract.

In hormone therapy users, the type of estrogen and/or progestin is documented, as is compliance, as missed tablets or nonadherence to patches may lead to irregular bleeding. The date and result of the last cervical Papanicolau smear, human papillomavirus (HPV) status, previous cervical smear abnormalities, coloposcopies, or cervical surgery should be reviewed and recorded.

A history of coagulation disorders should be elicited. Frequent intake of aspirin, nonsteroidal anti-inflammatory drugs, or other medications that inactivate platelet function should be noted. Iatrogenic anticoagulation has been shown to increase blood loss. Although only a small proportion of postmenopausal bleeding is attributed to anticoagulant medications, these patients pose a particular challenge as the diagnosis may not be realized and a woman may not respond to conventional treatments to stop endometrial bleeding.

Infection of the upper or lower genital tract can lead to abnormal bleeding in women of any age. Sexual activity and frequency should be elicited. Cervicitis, which may be caused by *Chlamydia* or gonorrhea, although uncommon in postmenopausal women, is possible and may cause irregular bleeding or postcoital spotting.

The clinician should explore the woman's perspective of her symptoms. By discussing her concerns, the clinician can ensure that she understands the process of diagnosis, treatments offered, expected outcomes, risks, and prognosis, as well as her prescriptives for therapy and follow-up.

Laboratory screening includes assessment for anemia, thyroid disease, and clotting disorders. Abdominal palpation may detect an enlarged fibroid uterus or abdominal mass. Inspection of the vulva and vagina is essential to exclude any gross pathology such as vulvar atrophy, abnormal growths, or vulvar dermatologic conditions.

> ### ☆ TIPS AND TRICKS
>
> Examination of the genital tract may reveal the level of estrogen exposure. A pale pink, dry, atrophic vagina with little or no cervical mucus indicates a chronic hypoestrogenic state. A moist, dark pink vagina with

rugations indicates an estrogenic state, especially if clear cervical mucus is identified. A simple saline vaginal wet preparation can further elucidate estrogen exposure. Alternately, a Papanicolau smear can be sent for cytologic evaluation of the "maturation index." Small parabasal cells with plump, noncondensed nuclei are seen with estrogen deficiency; large mature, cornified squamous cells with folded edges and small picnotic nuclei indicate estrogen exposure.

Speculum examination of the cervix excludes exocervical polyps or a macroscopic cervical tumor. Papanicolau smear screening is done if clinically indicated by the presence of a visible lesion or if a woman is due for a routine cervical cytology examination. Colposcopy should be done if any gross cervical lesion is noted. Vaginal and cervical swabs should be taken for gonorrhea and *Chlamydia* screening, as well as a saline wet preparation when a discharge is present or infection is suspected. The speculum should be rotated to view the entire vagina as lesions may be obscured by the anterior or posterior blade. The anus is inspected for fissures or external hemorrhoids.

The bimanual pelvic examination allows for assessment of uterine size and mobility, detection of pelvic tenderness, or palpation of an adnexal mass. Rectovaginal examination is done to palpate for cul-de-sac lesions and to confirm the bimanual examination. Palpate for hemorrhoids or anal lesions, and sample stool for occult blood.

Initial work-up

The diagnostic goal with postmenopausal bleeding is to exclude cancer and to identify underlying pathology to allow optimal treatment. TVUS has changed the evaluation of women with postmenopausal bleeding. Endometrial biopsy, hysteroscopy and targeted biopsy, or dilatation and curettage (D&C) is used when histologic sampling is needed. Diagnostic algorithms of postmenopausal bleeding focus on the identification of endometrial cancer as 90% of women with this cancer present with postmenopausal bleeding.

Laboratory studies may include a hemogram to evaluate anemia and the degree of blood loss in women with postmenopausal bleeding, and iron supplements prescribed as needed. The full blood count provides information about the platelet count and thereby identifies women with thrombocytopenia. Thyroid function tests (thyroid-stimulating hormone and free thyroxine) are indicated in women with symptoms of hypothyroidism including cold intolerance and fatigue, a family history of thyroid dysfunction, an abnormal thyroid examination, or if no testing has been done in last 3 years. Coagulation screening with a prothrombin time and partial thromboplastin time and clotting time may be indicated where there is a history of easy bruising, dental bleeding, menorrhagia since menarche, and a personal or family history suggesting a coagulation disorder. Follicle-stimulating hormone levels are not diagnostic of menopause.

> ### ★ TIPS AND TRICKS
>
> Cervical, endometrial, and other reproductive tract cancers can cause abnormal bleeding, and evidence for these tumors is sometimes found with Papanicolau smear screening. The most frequent abnormal cytologic results involve squamous cell pathology and may reflect cervicitis, intraepithelial neoplasia, or cancer. Less commonly, atypical glandular or endometrial cells may be found. Any of these may suggest the cause of bleeding, and, depending on the cytologic results, colposcopy or endometrial biopsy or both may be indicated.

Assessment of the uterine cavity (Figure 11.1)

Endometrial assessment in the patient with postmenopausal bleeding includes both structural and histologic abnormalities. The endometrial assessment may be by TVUS, endometrial biopsy, D&C, hysteroscopy and targeted biopsies, or magnetic resonance imaging (MRI). These modalities may be used in isolation or in combination.